Life and Death Decisions

Life and Death Decisions

Psychological and Ethical Considerations in End-of-Life Care

Phillip M. Kleespies

AMERICAN PSYCHOLOGICAL ASSOCIATION

WASHINGTON, DC

Published by
American Psychological Association
750 First Street, NE
Washington, DC 20002
www.apa.org

To order
APA Order Department
P.O. Box 92984
Washington, DC 20090-2984

Tel: (800) 374-2721; Direct: (202) 336-5510
Fax: (202) 336-5502; TDD/TTY: (202) 336-6123
Online: www.apa.org/books/
E-mail: order@apa.org

In the U.K., Europe, Africa, and the Middle East, copies may be ordered from
American Psychological Association
3 Henrietta Street
Covent Garden, London
WC2E 8LU England

Typeset in Goudy by MacAllister Publishing Services, Indianapolis, IN

Printer: Edwards Brothers, Inc., Ann Arbor, MI
Cover Designer: NiDesign, Baltimore, MD
Project Manager: MacAllister Publishing Services, Indianapolis, IN

The opinions and statements published are the responsibility of the author, and such opinions and statements do not necessarily represent the policies of the American Psychological Association.

Library of Congress Cataloging-in-Publication Data
Kleespies, Phillip M.
    Life and death decisions : psychological and ethical considerations in
    end-of-life care / Phillip M. Kleespies.— 1st ed.
        p. cm.
    Includes bibliographical references and index.
    ISBN 1-59147-067-6 (hardcover : alk. paper)
        1. Terminal care—Moral and ethical aspects. 2. Terminal
    care—Psychological aspects. I. Title.
    R726.8.K565 2003
    179.7—dc21   2003008745

British Library Cataloguing-in-Publication Data
A CIP record is available from the British Library.

Printed in the United States of America
First Edition

This book is dedicated to my mother, Tillie,
and to my mother-in-law, Rose,
both of whom lived to a great age and died
a modern death as I wrote it.

Oh as I was young and easy in the mercy of his means,
Time held me green and dying
Though I sang in my chains like the sea.

—Dylan Thomas, *Fern Hill*, l. 52–54

CONTENTS

PREFACE

My interest in the topic of end-of-life decisions grew out of my work on a previous book, *Emergencies in Mental Health Practice: Evaluation and Management* (Kleespies, 1998). One of the behavioral emergencies discussed was patients' suicidal behavior. One cannot think much about the topic of suicide without wondering why some people care so little for life or feel so miserable that they destroy themselves, while others are so resilient and invested in living that they will tolerate all manner of trials and tribulations to maintain themselves. This same topic is played out in bold relief among terminally ill patients in our current era, for most of us now die slowly of progressive and debilitating illnesses that can gradually corrode the human spirit and lay waste to human dignity. Faced with such conditions, some who are dying have longed for a hastened death, while others have longed for maximum curative efforts despite the apparent futility of the situation.

While working on *Emergencies in Mental Health Practice*, I had the opportunity to join the Ethics Advisory Committee (EAC) of the VA Boston Healthcare System. Participation as a member of the EAC has, in turn, presented me with the opportunity to think about and struggle with many of the ethical issues encountered in end-of-life care. Subsequent contact with members of American Psychological Association's (APA's) Ad Hoc Committee on End-of-Life Issues heightened my awareness of the fact that relatively few psychologists have been involved in clinical work with terminally ill patients or as members of hospital ethics advisory committees in which issues related to these patients are discussed. In fact, the Ad Hoc Committee and its predecessor, the APA Working Group on Assisted Suicide and End-of-Life Decisions (2000), have been of the opinion that psychology has been relatively invisible among the disciplines involved in end-of-life care as well as in the national debate that continues today about issues such as hastening death, assisted suicide, futility of treatment, and the rationing of scarce medical resources.

This book is about the choices that people have in regard to how they will die and the ways psychologists can help patients, families, healthcare proxies, and healthcare systems make those choices in humane and ethical ways. Although I have written this book primarily with the psychologist in mind, all the issues discussed are pertinent to other mental health and health practitioners such as social workers, nurses, and physicians. In writing this book, I have attempted to present a realistic rather than a romanticized version of our end-of-life options and the constraints on them. Thus, although self-determination and dignity during the process of dying may be highly valued by many in our society, they are often severely limited by the ravages of illness. Hopefully, clinicians who have become informed and sensitized to the pertinent issues will not be deterred. They will do all that they can to palliate suffering and foster an ending to life that is consistent with the values of the dying person.

ACKNOWLEDGMENTS

I am grateful for the opportunity to have been a member of the Ethics Advisory Committee (EAC) of the VA Boston Healthcare System. It is as a member of the EAC that I have encountered the cases that give meaning to this work. The life and death struggles of patients who are terminally ill, the trials of their families and surrogates, and the discussions with colleagues on the EAC have challenged, stimulated, and enriched my thinking. I would particularly like to thank two members of the EAC, Michele J. Karel, PhD, and the late Margaret W. Berrio, RN, MHA (EAC cochair), who took the time and effort to review and critique the first draft of each chapter of this book. I am very grateful to them for their contributions. Tragically, Margaret (Marge) Berrio died suddenly, and prematurely by modern standards, while this book was under review. It is ironic that such a guardian of patient autonomy should die with so very little choice in the time and manner of her death. As cochair of the EAC, Marge was a strong advocate for ethical approaches to end-of-life care. Her leadership, dedication, hard work, educative efforts, and obvious love of life are sorely missed.

I should note that the views and opinions expressed in this book are mine and do not necessarily represent the views and opinions of the EAC of the VA Boston Healthcare System or of the Veterans Health Administration.

I am particularly indebted to James L. Werth Jr., PhD, for the time and effort that he put into a comprehensive and detailed peer review. His comments and suggestions have been invaluable. Special thanks also to William E. Haley, PhD, who generously allowed me to read and cite an as yet unpublished manuscript that he and others from the American Psychological Association's (APA's) Ad Hoc Committee on End-of-Life Issues had written on clinical roles for psychologists in end-of-life care. In addition, my thanks to Vanessa Downing, the APA development editor, for her excellent review, and to Susan Reynolds, APA senior acquisitions editor, who originally suggested that I write this book and who provided support throughout the publication process.

Finally, I would like to thank my wife, Penelope, for her patience during the long hours that I devoted to writing this book and for her willingness to be a sounding board as I experimented with various ideas related to it.

Life and Death Decisions

INTRODUCTION

Knight: Who are you?

Death: I am death.

Knight: You have come for me?

Death: I have been a long time at your side.

Knight: That I know.

Death: Are you prepared?

Knight: My body is, but I am not.

> —*The Seventh Seal*, 1. 3-9, a film by Ingmar Bergman,
> original Swedish language version, subtitled in English

Psychosocial issues (e.g., a loss of perceived self-worth, a loss of independent functioning, depression, anxiety, hopelessness, social isolation, and poor quality of life) are frequently present among those with terminal illnesses whose ability to function is diminishing. Yet much of the research literature has primarily emphasized the physical aspects (i.e., the treatment of pain, nausea, vomiting, etc.) of caring for the dying (Emanuel & Emanuel, 1998; Werth, Gordon, & Johnson, 2002). Psychosocial issues rather than physical pain and discomfort, however, have been found to be the most frequent reasons given by people who request a hastened death (Breitbart, Rosenfeld, & Passik, 1996; Ganzini et al., 2000). It would seem reasonably clear, then, that a comprehensive approach to care for the terminally ill should include an effort to address the psychological, interpersonal, social, cultural, and spiritual needs of the patient. Some (e.g., those involved in the hospice movement) have endeavored to heighten awareness of the psychosocial needs of the dying (Butterfield-Picard & Magno, 1982), but there can be little doubt that a great need exists for others to contribute their expertise in order to reach a better resolution of this serious problem.

The discipline of psychology would seem to be a prime candidate for such a task. As noted in the preface to this volume, however, the American Psychological Association's Working Group on Assisted Suicide and End-of-Life Issues (2000) has concluded that "there is little evidence that the discipline of psychology as a whole has considered end-of-life issues to be an important area that deserves substantial professional time and attention" (p. 15). The Working Group arrived at this conclusion after investigating whether any substantial psychology activity regarding end-of-life issues existed in several domains (e.g., in curricula in undergraduate and graduate programs, in generating policies and guidelines for care, in testifying before legislative committees, in presentations at the annual APA convention and other meetings, and in publications in the major APA journals). By all these measures, psychology's relative lack of activity was considered noteworthy. Beyond this situation, however, or perhaps as a result of it, the Working Group found evidence that other health professions had not recognized psychology as an important discipline in the area of end-of-life practice. In this regard, for example, they cited the report of the Institute of Medicine on improving end-of-life care (Field & Cassel, 1997). Psychosocial care for the dying was discussed in this extensive report, but no mention was made of psychologists or psychiatrists as potential members of interdisciplinary palliative care teams. Rather, potential team members were seen as physicians, nurses, social workers, pharmacists, and chaplains.

The Working Group, as well as APA's more recently formed Ad Hoc Committee on End-of-Life Issues, has strongly recommended efforts to develop roles for psychologists in end-of-life care and in the ongoing national debate about end-of-life choices. This book has been written to try to further these objectives. It has a primary focus on ethical concerns and dilemmas, and the application of ethical principles to end-of-life decision making since these principles are fundamental to practice in an area where there can be deeply held and emotion-laden convictions on both sides of an issue.

In chapter 1, "Modern End-of-Life Issues: An Overview," the reasons for the major dilemmas that confront the terminally ill in the modern era are discussed. Advances in medicine, technology, and public health have led to greater longevity. The consequential increased frequency of prolonged death by degenerative disease, however, has brought with it concerns about quality of life for the dying and questions about whether death with dignity is possible. These concerns and issues have driven efforts by some to increase self-determination and control of the timing and circumstances of death. Yet the promise of modern medicine and technology seems to have led others to the belief that cure is always close at hand and that curative efforts should be continued despite sound medical opinions that they will be ineffective. This book is organized around these two major positions, which seem to be differing responses to the same phenomenon, that is, our increased ability to sustain life in the modern era.

Chapter 2, "Ethical and Legal Issues in End-of-Life Decisions," provides essential background information about the major ethical principles that guide the process of end-of-life decision making. It also presents the legal bases for many end-of-life decisions such as decisions to refuse life-sustaining treatment or decisions that may indirectly hasten death. In addition, it discusses the legal theory of informed consent and the criteria that have been proposed for determining one of the key elements of informed consent, that is, decision-making capacity or competency.

Chapter 3, "The Wish to Die: Decisions That Do Not Prolong or May Hasten the Dying Process," and chapter 4, "The Wish to Die: Assisted Suicide and Voluntary Euthanasia," explore the efforts of those who have sought greater self-determination in the process of dying. Chapter 3 specifically deals with those generally accepted healthcare practices that allow the patient some choice in the manner and timing of his or her death. These practices include decisions about withholding or withdrawing life-sustaining treatment, decisions in which a so-called *double effect* takes place (i.e., decisions in which death is not the primary intent, but the indirect result of attempts to provide relief of pain and suffering), and procedures that allow the patient to extend his or her right to make end-of-life choices to a time when he or she is no longer capable of informed decision making. Chapter 4, on the other hand, examines those more controversial practices, assisted suicide and voluntary euthanasia, that have not been widely accepted and are the subject of heated national debate.

Chapter 5, "The Wish to Prolong Life," takes up the issues confronted by terminally ill patients who, rather than wanting to have life come to an end, wish to prolong it for as long as possible. The major conflicts that these individuals encounter have to do with (a) requests for treatment when the healthcare staff believes that it will not be of benefit (i.e., the issue of so-called *futile treatment*), and (b) the problem of obtaining access to scarce resources for highly specialized life-sustaining treatments or procedures (i.e., the issue of *rationing*). The chapter also discusses the related issue of inequities in access to potentially life-sustaining treatments and to healthcare in general.

Chapter 6, "Alternatives in Care Near the End of Life," presents the major systems of care that are available near the end of life and discusses the settings in which people most frequently die. The potential choices of conventional medical care versus hospice care or palliative care are discussed, as well as the way in which these systems of care may intersect with the hospital, nursing home, or home setting for death. Finally, the chapter describes a new approach to care at the level of advanced illness but prior to terminal illness. The goal of this approach is to help the patient confront the seriousness of his or her illness and begin to formulate what preferences in care he or she might want as the illness progresses.

Chapter 7, "The Psychologist's Role in End-of-Life Care," is concerned with the need for psychologists to become more involved in addressing the psychological suffering and psychosocial needs of the terminally ill. It outlines the roles that they may fill in four time periods: (a) prior to progressive and life-threatening illness, (b) during the period of advanced illness, (c) when the patient's condition is terminal, and (d) during the period of bereavement (Haley, Niemeyer, Larson, Kwilosz, & Kasl-Godley, 2003). The chapter also discusses the potential role of psychologists on interdisciplinary teams (e.g., hospice or palliative care teams) and on committees such as an ethics advisory committee.

The book comes to a close with chapter 8, "Concluding Thoughts on Suffering, Dying, and Choice." This brief chapter discusses the distinction between bodily pain and a person's suffering, the need to demythologize death and focus on a more realistic view of the dying process, and the importance of fostering a new *dignity-conserving* model of end-of-life care (Chochinov, 2002).

As one reads this book, it is important to keep in mind that the approach to end-of-life issues discussed in it is, in large measure, a product of the prevailing European American culture with which western medicine is heavily imbued (Hallenbeck, Goldstein, & Mebane, 1996). Yet our society is becoming increasingly diverse and multicultural, and many patients and families do not share the dominant culture's values and meanings with regard to death and dying. Thus, for example, informing the patient fully about his or her condition is considered an obligation of clinical staff in the American medical system. It has, in fact, been codified in the doctrine of informed consent that states, in part, that we must be sure that the patient understands his or her condition and the treatment that is being proposed. Yet in some non-European American and Native American cultures, strong prohibitions exist against such full disclosure (Werth, Blevins, Toussaint, & Durham, 2002). In effect, family members may be expected to protect the individual from bad news and to help him or her sustain hope. With such patients and families, the potential for cross-cultural misunderstanding and insensitivity seems clear.

For those in the United States who work with the dying, it is important to emphasize what Hern, Koenig, Moore, and Marshall (1998) have stated: "that culture is not simply an inconvenient barrier to a rational, scientifically based healthcare system" (p. 31). Rather, respect for the culturally based values of the dying person and his or her family can be crucial to what the patient and family consider a dignified death. Recognizing and working with such differences can be challenging, but Hern et al. have offered a model for doing so that involves discussion and an effort to explain the values inherent in the ethical principles espoused by American medicine.

The first step is listening to the patient's and the family's thoughts about the patient's illness and its seriousness. Once some understanding of the patient's personal and cultural perspective is attained, an effort can be made to explain the value that the predominant system of bioethics has placed on such issues as informing patients about their illness and treatment options. This explanation might include stating how the intent of informed consent is to respect the person and to protect him or her from harm and unwanted treatment. It also would include a discussion of how not informing the patient might run counter to the principles of the healthcare system and the end-of-life care team. The patient, the family, and the clinician can then negotiate what level of involvement, if any, the patient will find comfortable. As Hern et al. have pointed out, such an offer of informed consent, at the least, respects the patient's right to information even if the patient chooses to remain relatively uninformed.

Of course, religious beliefs and spirituality, in addition to cultural values, are also sources of purpose and meaning for many people. Such beliefs can become increasingly so as purpose and meaning are tested by the approach of life's end. For those who are dying, it is believed that religion and faith in a divine being can sometimes mediate the quality of life by enhancing the patient's sense of security and well-being (Daaleman & VandeCreek, 2000). This book has not been written from a particular religious or spiritual perspective, but it does recognize that different religious and spiritual points of view on death and dying need to be acknowledged and respected. Some of the opinions and positions expressed in this book may, at times, be dissonant with particular religious and spiritual beliefs and values. I would like to acknowledge that such differences in point of view often exist in our society and need to be carefully taken into consideration when approaching end-of-life care and decision making.

1

MODERN END-OF-LIFE ISSUES: AN OVERVIEW

In recent generations, we have added something new: We have created the method of modern dying. Modern dying takes place in the modern hospital, where it can be hidden, cleansed of its organic blight, and finally packaged for modern burial. We can now deny the power not only of death but of nature itself.

—Nuland, 1995, p. xv

Mr. J was a 55-year-old, married, successful business executive who had had only minor health problems in his life. His children were grown and living independently. After years of child rearing, he and his wife now had additional leisure time. They had begun to take more frequent weekend trips and vacations. They enjoyed the occasional local drama production, and they often spent a Sunday afternoon at the art museum. On one particular Sunday, as they were in line awaiting entry into one of the museum's exhibits, disaster seemed to strike. Mr. J began to feel weak and sweaty. Then he felt a constricting pressure in his chest that radiated down his left arm. Suddenly, the pressure became incredibly intense. He grasped his chest with both hands and fell to the floor unable to breathe. His face became blue and swollen.

Mr. J's wife shouted for help. Several museum staff members came running. A year before, the museum had all of its staff trained in cardiopulmonary resuscitation (CPR). A staff member quickly checked to see if Mr. J had an open airway. He listened for respirations and felt Mr. J's neck for a pulse. There was none. He started chest compressions while a second staff member started mouth-to-mouth resuscitation. Mr. J was fortunate. He started to breathe again. An ambulance was called, and Mr. J was rapidly transported to a nearby emergency room where his condition was stabilized; later that day he was admitted to a cardiac intensive care unit.

During Mr. J's hospital stay, he had a number of medical tests, including an angiogram. It was determined that he had a significant occlusion of his coronary arteries and that he was at grave risk of future heart attacks. Triple bypass surgery was recommended and performed and he left the hospital with a heart whose functioning was much improved. He gradually resumed his life and worked productively for another 10 years before retiring. Mr. J never suffered another heart attack. Because of the occlusion of smaller coronary vessels, his heart needed to work harder and gradually weakened. His circulation became sluggish, as did the functioning of his lungs. He was put on oxygen and given a portable tank, but he did not like feeling tethered to an oxygen tank and having decreased mobility. Even with the use of continuous oxygen, his breathing eventually became very labored. He died, not very comfortably, of chronic congestive heart failure and pneumonia.

This case scenario illustrates some of the remarkable advances in medicine and medical technology that have radically changed life expectancy and patterns of death and dying during the 20th century, and that promise to continue to do so into the 21st century. Pertinent to this case, Nuland (1993) has noted that the death rate from heart attacks has decreased by approximately 30% in the past three decades, while mortality from congestive heart failure has increased by one third.

In this chapter, we discuss how advances in managing and treating acute, life-threatening illnesses have not only led to greater longevity and hopefulness but also seem to have brought about a lengthening of the typical dying trajectory and, on average, a more prolonged period of disability. An extended period of disability and dying raises questions about quality of life in its final phases and whether the notion of death with dignity is realistic. These questions are also discussed.

One central thesis of the chapter (and of the book) is that people's concern about the prospect of such prolonged, medicalized, often impersonal, and, at times, agonizing deaths is driving them to try to establish a greater degree of self-determination in the dying process. Whether economic concerns about the cost of end-of-life care may confound this proposition is also examined.

A second major thesis is that the same progress in biomedical science that has been successful in prolonging life (and the so-called living-dying interval) has also contributed to an intensified belief of many that medical research and continued efforts at treatment will always lead to the cure for an individual's disease or injury, even in the face of predictions that further treatment is *futile* or will only lead to greater suffering. Such a belief has arisen not only from the fact that the human race has always longed for continued life, if not immortality, but because advances of biomedical science in the modern era seem to have fueled the mythology that the defeat of disease and the restoration of health are just a step away. When death is near, then, it seems that many in our society struggle with the two sides of this existential dilemma, that is, whether to fight on strenuously with the hope of a reprieve if not a cure, or to attempt to bow out gracefully with the acknowledgment that meaningful life is essentially over.

INCREASING LONGEVITY

Seale (2000) has pointed out that the average life expectancy at birth worldwide has risen from 48 years in 1955 to 65 years in 1995. In developed countries like the United States, the average life expectancy has increased from approximately 47 years in 1900 to a record high of 76.7 years in 1998, an increase of nearly 30 years (National Center for Health Statistics, 2000). Women in the United States can now, on average, expect to live to age 79, and men to age 73 (Wehrwein, 1999). The percentage of the population that is 65 years of age and older has been steadily rising. It has been said that the most rapidly growing age group in the United States is centenarians. In 1950, there were approximately 4,475 people who were 100 years of age or older, while by 1990, the number had increased to approximately 54,000 (Walker & Charlton, 1999).

Although these gains are spectacular, at least two points are particularly noteworthy. One is that, if taken at face value, these gains are at risk of masking an unevenness both within and across countries; another is that increases in life expectancy have slowed down. Within the United States and across race–gender groups, for example, White females have the highest life expectancy at birth (i.e., 79.9 years), while African American males have the lowest at 67.2 years. On average, the White population in the United States currently lives 6.0 years longer than African Americans (Centers for Disease Control, 1999), while in England, Melzer, McWilliams, Brayne, Johnson, and Bond (2000) have reported that an overall pattern of significantly higher rates of morbidity and mortality exists in the less privileged social classes.

When comparing developed countries with other regions of the world, the differences are more pronounced. Mainly as a result of the AIDS epidemic, life expectancy in sub-Saharan Africa is reportedly falling to "medieval" levels. In Uganda, for example, life expectancy at birth in 1995–2000 was only 41.4 years (Seale, 2000). Meanwhile, in Russia, it has been reported that life expectancy for males dropped from 64.3 years in 1985–1990 to 57.5 years in 1994. Middle-aged Russian males seem to have been most affected by increased deaths from cardiovascular disease, accidental poisoning, suicide, and, most striking, by homicide.

As noted earlier, gains continue to be made in the average life expectancy in the United States, but the rate of increase has diminished. Actually, the largest gains occurred before 1950 with the reduction of infant and early childhood mortality rates and with the introduction of antibiotics and vaccines that reduced the risk of death from infectious diseases. Despite the losses suffered in World War I, the decade with the largest increase was 1910–1920, which saw a rise in life expectancy at birth of 5 years. The rate of increase slowed to approximately 1.5 years by the decade 1980–1990 (Seale, 2000; Wehrwein, 1999).

It is well-known that the increase in life expectancy in developed countries such as the United States, Japan, and many European nations has to do with changes in the causes of death. Despite the many problems with the health care system in countries like the United States, advances in medicine and public health are more readily available than in developing countries. As a result, infectious diseases have diminished in importance as causes of death, and degenerative diseases have become the major causes of death (Seale, 2000). Epidemics from diseases such as diphtheria, whooping cough, and smallpox have caused large numbers of deaths in the past. Because infants in most developed countries are now routinely vaccinated against these diseases, the degenerative diseases that occur more frequently in adulthood, such as cancer, heart disease, and stroke, have emerged as the leading causes of death.

Advances in the treatment of degenerative diseases have been slower and more difficult to achieve. This, of course, is not to say that progress has not been made. The bypass surgery in the case noted at the beginning of the chapter is a clear example of a modern surgical procedure that has prolonged the lives of many victims of coronary artery disease. Nor is it to say that there will not be future biomedical breakthroughs that vastly alter the course of dying by degenerative disease. Witness, for example, the current testing of new classes of drugs like endostatin and angiostatin that may be able to cut off the blood supply and "starve" cancerous tumors.

Moreover, speculation exists about how the body itself may be able to repair damage done by disease and aging. In this regard, Harris (2000), for example, has suggested that cloned human embryonic stem cells might be reprogrammed and used for the regeneration of organs and tissues and that genes that contribute to certain diseases and to aging might be rendered ineffective in the early embryonic stages. Harris (1998) believes that we are on the verge of a revolution in molecular biology and genetics that could be of tremendous power in terms of its potential to alter genetic coding for antibodies against major infections and for enzymes that could destroy carcinogens. Significantly extended average life expectancy would clearly accompany such progress in biomedical science and biotechnology.

As interesting, exciting, and, in some respects, disconcerting as such possibilities may be, they are clearly not here yet. Rather, as Nuland (1993) has pointed out, our current situation is that we have increased our average life expectancy, but "the maximum has not changed in verifiable recorded history" (p. 85). He argues for a species-determined limit to life spans, and, in man, it does not exceed 120 years at its longest. From this perspective, life has natural, inherent limits, and even in the absence of disease or an accident, the trajectory of life will reach an end. In Nuland's terms, "the very old do not succumb to disease—they implode their way into eternity" (p. 83). Unless or until the revolution in genetics predicted by Harris (1998) occurs, these apparent limits of life spans seem to be what we can expect.

PROLONGED DYING AND CONCERNS ABOUT QUALITY OF LIFE

High-profile cases like those of Karen Ann Quinlan (*In re Quinlan*, 1976) and Nancy Beth Cruzan (*Cruzan v. Director, Missouri Department of Health*, 1990) brought to public attention the fact that medical technology had advanced to the point where it could sustain life even when the individual was in a persistent state of unconsciousness with no hope of recovery. Karen Quinlan, who at the age of 20 suffered irreversible brain damage, was kept alive in a comatose state on a respirator for years. Her emaciated body was routinely turned and attended by nursing staff. At that time (in the mid-1970s), her doctors were unwilling to disconnect her from the respirator despite her family's repeated requests that she be allowed to die. Her father was eventually able to obtain court authority to refuse unwanted medical treatment (i.e., mechanical ventilation) on his daughter's behalf. However, she lingered for 8 years while receiving artificial nutrition and hydration. The apparent meaninglessness of such an existence without consciousness, and the reluctance of the medical community and the state to allow such an individual to die, set off alarms about the loss of self-determination and personal control over conditions at the end of life. In the wake of court decisions such as those in the cases of *Quinlan* and others (e.g., *Cruzan*), medical staff are no longer so reluctant to withdraw or withhold life-sustaining treatment under similar circumstances. Other factors, however, have continued to drive the national concern over control of the dying process.

In an era when epidemics could sweep across the country and medical technology was still relatively primitive, dying was often comparatively rapid. The time and opportunity for choices that might influence how one dies were likely to be limited. A prevailing fear was that there would be no possibility for reconciliation, closure, or the chance to say farewell. Such sudden or rapid death has by no means been eradicated. People still die of heart attacks, strokes, accidental injuries, homicides, suicides, and so forth. With the medical advances noted above, however, the developed countries have reached the point where 70% to 80% of people now die later in life and slowly of degenerative disease rather than of acute disease or injury (Liao, McGee, Cao, & Cooper, 2000). Now, one can live for years with a disease that kills one little by little (American Geriatrics Society, 1997). Seale (2000) has observed that, although average life expectancy has increased, so-called healthy life expectancy (i.e., years of life in good health or without significant disability) has not.

The prospect of a prolonged and slow dying process from illnesses that can deprive the individual of autonomy and dignity has continued to fuel concerns in a significant segment of our society about the quality of life in its final phases. The possibility of living to the point of suffering from dementia with associated mental confusion, loss of memory, and a greatly reduced ability to recognize and interact with loved ones has deeply concerned many. In addition, a heightened awareness has arisen that prolonged and debilitating deaths often become "medicalized;"that is, they occur in hospitals and nursing homes with attendant medical procedures that also affect privacy, autonomy, and dignity.

QUALITY OF LIFE AT THE END OF LIFE

"They take us here. They take us there. They keep us locked up. I don't belong here." These are the words of an elderly woman who has Parkinson's disease and resides in a nursing home. They reflect the fear that people may have about the effects of a progressive and debilitating illness in old age, that one will lose the ability to make choices and exercise control over one's life. Her comments also seem to suggest another fear: a loss of meaning and purpose. This woman's circumstances are not uncommon in modern America; those with advanced illness and terminal illness often reside in hospitals and nursing homes. Such institutional care, although by no means universal in the United States, has been increasingly adopted as a solution to the decreased availability of informal care for the elderly in families (Seale, 2000). It is estimated that 70% to 80% of deaths in developed countries like the United States and Britain now occur in hospitals and other institutions (Black & Jolley, 1990; Nuland, 1993).

Partly as a result of such developments, quality of life has emerged in the past 20 to 30 years as an important consideration in decisions about end-of-life care. Hundreds if not thousands of studies and articles have been published on this topic. Although such activity seems to represent a concerted effort, Gill and Feinstein (1994), after a critical review of the literature, stated, "Despite the proliferation of instruments and the burgeoning theoretical literature devoted to the measurement of quality of life, no unified approach has been devised for its measurement, and little agreement has been attained on what it means" (p. 619). These authors did several computer searches for articles on quality of life. From the hundreds of articles identified, they randomly selected 75. In only 11 articles in this sample was there an effort to define the concept of quality of life. In the 75 studies, a total of 159 different instruments were used to measure quality of life. Of these instruments, 136 were used in only one study. Although many of the studies used elegant and sophisticated statistical techniques, the authors ultimately questioned whether these techniques and approaches were satisfactory for determining what clinicians and patients perceive as quality of life. In effect, they have argued that quality of life is a uniquely personal perception and that measurement of it needs to be based on the distinctive thoughts, feelings, and values of the individuals involved.

In this regard, Gill and Feinstein also found that in the majority (i.e., 87%) of the studies they sampled, patients were not invited to add any individual responses but were permitted to respond only to those items selected by the *experts*. Moreover, in over 90% of the articles, patients were not even asked to rate or rank the importance of individual items for their quality of life. Cohen and colleagues (Cohen & Mount, 1992; Cohen, Mount, Tomas, & Mount, 1996) have also been sharply critical of many of the existing quality of life instruments. They have pointed out that most measures of quality of life have been weighted toward physical issues to the neglect of psychological issues, such as meaning and purpose. As they have noted, however, considerable physical suffering can be overridden by an increased sense of personal meaning, just as physical status can be adversely affected by a loss of purpose.

In an attempt to avoid the pitfalls of a strictly quantitative and physical-symptom-driven approach to measuring quality of life, two groups of investigators (Byock & Merriman, 1998; Cohen, Mount, Strobel, & Bui, 1995) have recently developed instruments that are more oriented to psychological and existential issues and to incorporating the reported experience of the patient. As Cohen et al. (1997) have pointed out, determining one's quality of life is a subjective matter and, like assessing pain, we are often in the position of accepting that it is what the person says it is. They have further noted that while patients' objectively observable status may suggest a low quality of life, they have frequently found that patients rate their own quality of life as more satisfactory than expert observers do. In effect, these investigators have challenged the notion that quality of life necessarily declines at the same rate as physical health.

For a more complete description of the quality of life instruments by Byock and Merriman (1998) and Cohen et al. (1995), refer to the Appendix at the end of this chapter. Additional information on quality of life instruments can also be obtained from the Toolkit of Instruments to Measure End-of-Life Care Web site (www.chcr.brown.edu/pcoc/toolkit.htm), published by the Center for Gerontology and Health Care Research at Brown Medical School (2000, October 1).

QUALITY END-OF-LIFE CARE

Modern medicine, with all of its impressive array of technologically sophisticated equipment and procedures, is deeply and primarily committed to saving and sustaining life. As Sherwin Nuland (1993) has stated it,

> The quest of every doctor in approaching serious disease is to make the diagnosis and design and carry out the specific cure. This quest, I call The Riddle, and I capitalize it so there is no mistaking its dominance over every other consideration. The satisfaction of solving The Riddle is its own reward, and the fuel that drives the clinical engines of medicine's most highly trained specialists. It is every doctor's measure of his own abilities; it is the most important ingredient in his professional self-image. (p. 248)

For reasons such as these, it has been difficult for those in medicine and related disciplines to refocus on end-of-life care, that is, on care that is not directed toward a cure and the restoration of functions, but toward palliation or the reduction of the intensity of suffering in someone who is, in fact, dying. It is encouraging, however, that recent efforts have been made to identify what might constitute quality of care for those who are at the end of life.

To this end, the American Geriatrics Society has published a document entitled "Measuring Quality of Care at the End of Life: A Statement of Principles" (1997). It was endorsed not only by the American Geriatrics Society but also by 40 other organizations, among them the American Cancer Society, the American Medical Association, and the American Nurses Association. The document has articulated 10 domains to be considered when evaluating quality of care at the end of life. They include (a) physical and emotional symptom management, (b) support of function and autonomy, (c) advance care planning, (d) careful consideration of the wisdom of aggressive care near death, (e) patient and family satisfaction with the care given, (f) the individual's global quality of life, (g) the financial and emotional burden on the family, (h) health care pressures to accept death too readily, (i) continuity of care, and the skill of care providers, and (j) the bereavement of family members after the patient's death. The statement encourages funding organizations and researchers to develop the tools needed to measure quality of care for the terminally ill within this framework.

Others such as Field and Cassel (1997) and Emanuel and Emanuel (1998) have also provided frameworks (with slightly different areas of emphasis) for evaluating the quality of end-of-life care. Although these have all been thoughtful and worthy endeavors, Singer, Martin, and Kelner (1999) have pointed out that they were derived from the medical expert perspective rather than from the perspective of patients and their families. They have argued that the patient's and family's point of view belongs at the center of one's focus on what constitutes quality end-of-life care. This argument, of course, is analogous to that made by Gill and Feinstein (1994) in regard to the measurement of quality of life. Singer et al. (1999) analyzed data from three previous studies in which they had conducted in-depth, open-ended, face-to-face interviews with three groups of patients: dialysis patients, HIV-positive patients, and residents of a long-term care facility (Kelner, 1995; Martin, Thiel, & Singer, 2002; Singer et al., 1998). In general, the interviewers questioned participants about the content and process of their advance care planning and their views on control over decision making at the end of life. The responses were coded and labeled as specific end-of-life issues.

Through the above process, the investigators identified five domains of quality end-of-life care: (a) receiving adequate pain and symptom management, (b) avoiding inappropriate prolongation of dying, (c) achieving a sense of control over end-of-life decisions, (d) relieving the burden of their dying on loved ones, and (e) strengthening relationships with loved ones through communication about their dying. Compared with the expert-derived frameworks, the authors have pointed out that this patient-derived description of quality end-of-life care is simpler, more straightforward, and more specific. It omits vague concepts like global or overall quality of life. In addition, it has inherent authenticity. They recommended that these five domains be used as the conceptual foundation for research and practice in regard to what constitutes quality end-of-life care.

The expert-derived and the patient-derived frameworks have considerable overlap. Both have points that merit consideration by those who work with dying patients. Despite these efforts to define quality end-of-life care, however, real-life barriers to achieving it remain in place. As Zerzan, Stearns, and Hanson (2000) have pointed out, current health policy tends to discourage the use of palliative and hospice care for nursing home residents who are terminally ill. By and large, reimbursement rules provide incentives for restorative care and technologically intensive treatment rather than for labor-intensive palliative care. If a potential nursing home resident has only Medicare coverage and would like to have hospice care, Medicare will pay for hospice care, but the nursing home then receives less reimbursement and the resident must pay for room and board. As a result, many nursing homes do not offer hospice services under Medicare alone. Medical centers and hospitals are also reluctant to commit themselves to establishing palliative care units or programs that are less remunerative than acute treatment units. For these and other reasons, programs that focus on delivering quality end-of-life care have been less than optimally available.

IS DEATH WITH DIGNITY A MYTH?

Although improved quality of life for dying patients and quality end-of-life care are worthy pursuits in and of themselves, the hope is that they will culminate in the so-called good death or death with dignity. What exactly, however, is meant by *death with dignity*? For some, it might mean simply dying in peace or with relative peace of mind (Tobin, 1999). Others, such as Battin (1994), have made an effort to define more specifically, at least within the dominant European American culture in the United States, what may be meant by death with dignity. In general, she holds that it implies death with a sense of self-worth and self-respect. Yet, in particular, she has defined it as a term that refers to dying while still retaining those qualities that tend to give one a sense of worth and respect, that is, self-awareness, self-determination or the ability to make one's own decisions, self-acceptance, and the ability to take responsibility for one's own actions.

Of course, as noted in the next section of this chapter, such a definition does not apply to all in a pluralistic society. Nonetheless, Nuland (1993) has contended that this dominant culture's ideal of death with dignity has increasingly become a myth in the modern era. Thus, he has noted that

> . . . the belief in the probability of death with dignity is our, and society's, attempt to deal with the reality of what is all too frequently a series of destructive events that involve by their very nature the disintegration of the dying person's humanity. I have not often seen much dignity in the process by which we die. (p. xvii)

Nuland, a surgeon who has seen death close up, has a dark but perhaps realistic vision; it is, to some degree, supported by Battin (1994) who has maintained that, under current conditions, the best that the terminally ill patient can hope for is "the least worst death among those that could naturally occur" (p. 36). Likewise, Emanuel and Emanuel 1998 have noted that we face a paradox in which increased concern surrounds how we die and a tremendous ability to relieve symptoms and improve care exists, yet persistent suffering is experienced by many dying patients. Perspectives such as these have been supported by the findings of the SUPPORT Principal Investigators (1995) in their large, multisite study of care for the seriously ill. These findings suggest that modern dying is often far from the longed-for peaceful and serene passage in which one is surrounded and comforted by loving family and friends, as it is sometimes portrayed in the literature (e.g., Tobin, 1999).

As with the term death with dignity, the concept of *natural death* has also taken on a romanticized connotation (Battin, 1994). In earlier struggles to avoid a technologically prolonged death, proponents of the right-to-die movement advocated for what was referred to as natural death, or the right to die under conditions that were relatively free of invasive medical procedures and, at times, noxious treatments. In some states such as California and North Carolina, laws that were referred to as natural death laws were enacted. As Battin (1994) and Kleespies and Mori (1998) have pointed out, death under such circumstances was often envisioned as a peaceful, painless, technologically unencumbered, more humane process. No guarantee exists, however, that this will be the case. In fact, many natural deaths can be quite painful and far from peaceful. They may be less prolonged, but they are not necessarily easier.

The reality is that despite improvements in pain and symptom management, the dying process often involves considerable mental anguish and physical distress. Consider, for example, an elderly woman who is the resident of a nursing home and has severe emphysema. Her lungs have lost much of their elasticity. The struggle simply to breathe goes on every day. Although she is on continuous oxygen, any amount of exertion brings on episodes of air hunger in which she gasps for air and feels panicked about suffocating. When she is given anxiolytic medication to reduce her anxiety, she becomes mentally confused and distressed about her confusion. Her heart is strong, however, and she lives on in this condition for a year and a half. She can only manage to communicate on the simplest level. Visits from family members become less and less meaningful as her world constricts to simply surviving each day. Eventually, her condition worsens and she is heavily sedated with morphine to diminish her discomfort. Her heart finally gives out and her struggle is over. As Battin (1994) has pointed out, such a death hardly allows for the peaceful leave-taking imagined in the notion of natural death or death with dignity. As Nuland (1993) has said, "There is no dignity in this kind of death. It is an arbitrary act of nature and an affront to the humanity of its victims" (p. 117).

It is not that a relatively natural death might not be preferable or that we should cease to try to achieve death with dignity. Chochinov (2002), for example, has recently proposed an approach called *dignity-conserving care*, which includes having terminally ill people speak on tape about aspects of their lives that they would most want remembered. We need to be realistic, however, and accept that death with dignity is an ideal that may currently be attained to some degree by some and more fully by a few, but it is far from a certainty for all. If it is attained, it is typically through a collaborative effort on the part of the patient, the patient's family and friends, and the health care staff. If we expect that it will automatically be given to us, then we are indeed in the realm of myth and likely to leave life surprised and disappointed that such things could happen to us and to our loved ones. Likewise, if we were to naively choose a natural death free from all medical intervention, then we might deny ourselves those opportunities in which a minor procedure or intervention, although not curative, might nonetheless make the dying process easier. Thus, for example, a tumor in the intestinal tract of an otherwise terminally ill patient might be surgically removed to save the patient from the added suffering of distention, increased pain, vomiting, possible hemorrhage, and so forth. At times, nature may need some assistance if pain and suffering are to be kept at tolerable levels.

THE IDEAL OF DEATH WITH DIGNITY IN A DIVERSE SOCIETY

The concept of individual autonomy is highly valued in the United States. The origins of the country were based on it. The concept of death with dignity as articulated in the preceding section is pervaded by this individualistic approach, that is, by an emphasis on self-determination and individual responsibility as values. Yet as noted in the introduction to this volume, our culture has become increasingly diverse. It is, therefore, important to realize that, as the APA Working Group (2000) has pointed out, certain segments of the population, which have their own value systems, may not agree with the larger autonomy-focused discourse on death and dying.

The APA Working Group (2000) has articulated certain assumptions that underlie our orientation to individual autonomy with respect to end-of-life issues. These assumptions include the following: (a) that the individual is the primary decision-maker and wishes to be so, (b) that the individual has the personal power to make the choices he or she wants, (c) that the individual has equal financial access to different options, (d) that the individual values discussing and planning for death, (e) that clear communication and understanding exists between the individual and the health care team, and (f) that the individual's spiritual orientation allows for choice in the time and manner of death. Clearly, it is not safe to make such assumptions for all groups in our pluralistic society.

Hallenbeck, Goldstein, and Mebane (1996), for example, have discussed how immigrants or the children of immigrants from certain Asian cultures may not place the same value on individual autonomy as we do in the West. Rather, they may emphasize family role obligations. An elderly parent from such a cultural background might willingly cede decision-making authority to an adult son who is expected to use his judgment to protect the well-being of his parent. The son's focus may be less on the wishes of the parent as an individual, however, and more on fulfilling what he perceives as his familial and societal role.

As another example, the African American community has experienced unequal access to medical care, a situation that has raised doubts for them about the credibility of the health care system. Crawley et al. (2000) have contended that these circumstances may, in part, account for why African Americans are more likely to want to be kept alive on life support even when the effort seems relatively hopeless. Such circumstances may also explain the relatively diminished interest that they seem to have in discussing and completing advance directives. Thus, in a study comparing African Americans, Hispanics, and non-Hispanic Whites, African Americans were the most likely to feel that completing advance directives meant relinquishing control and could lead to less desirable care (Caralis, Davis, Wright, & Marcial, 1993).

Certain Native American groups like the Navajo people believe that thought and language have the power to shape reality. Their view is that health is restored through thinking and speaking in a positive way (Carrese & Rhodes, 1995). Advance care planning demands that patients think about their illness and the distinct possibility that it will worsen. In the Navajo culture, such planning would mean thinking in a negative way and could result in harm to the individual. It comes as no surprise, then, that in a series of in-depth interviews, Carrese and Rhodes found that the vast majority of Navajo participants felt that completing advance directives was a serious violation of their traditional values and ways of thinking.

Observations such as those just noted remind us that the moral concepts and principles of Western thought are not universally held even in our own country. What is considered a dignified death, and the course of attaining it, can also vary depending on the cultural background of the individual. We need to be aware of and respect the diverse ways in which people of different cultural, ethnic, or racial backgrounds may conceive of the dying process and the meaning of death with dignity (Hallenbeck et al., 1996). The meaning may not be as imbued with notions of autonomous decision making as mainstream U.S. culture.

SELF-DETERMINATION OR COST-CONTROLLED DYING?

The Patient Self-Determination Act (PSDA) of 1990 was widely hailed as an important affirmation of a patient's right to autonomous decision making with regard to his or her health care at the end of life, and so it was. The PSDA made it a requirement that hospitals, nursing homes, hospices, HMOs, and other health care facilities that take Medicaid or Medicare patients inform them of their right to accept or refuse medical or surgical treatment. Patients also had the right to formulate advance directives about their health care if they reach a stage when they are no longer capable of making their own decisions. As impressive as this legislation was, Battin (1994) has raised the question of whether it was also a "cloaked cost-control proposal" (p. 14).

Little doubt exists that health care spending in the United States is very high. As Field and Cassel (1997) have indicated, spending on care at the end of life is also quite high and is in large measure financed by government programs. Emanuel (1996) has pointed out that medical care at the end of life consumes 10% to 12% of the total U.S. health care budget, and 27% to 30% of Medicare payments each year go to the 5% to 6% of Medicare patients who die that year. In the effort to reduce overall health care expenditures, spending on end-of-life care has, in fact, attracted considerable attention as a possible source of savings. In particular, questions have been raised about whether a wider use of advance directives, more referrals to hospice and palliative care (with their emphasis on comfort measures as opposed to high-tech acute care), and the resultant reduction in so-called *futile* treatments for the terminally ill might lead to a reduction in overall health care cost.

Emanuel and Emanuel (1994) have attempted to estimate cost savings that the health care system might realize if it employed the means just mentioned. With regard to advance directives, the thinking has been that having an advance directive in which the patient states that he or she does not want heroic measures would diminish the medical profession's drive to use high-tech and costly efforts with patients who were unlikely to respond to such life-prolonging interventions (Field & Cassel, 1997).

Two retrospective, chart-based studies (Chambers, Diamond, Perkel, & Lasch, 1994; Weeks, Kofoed, Wallace, & Welch, 1994) found that the documentation of advance directives in the medical record was associated with great cost savings. In two studies that were prospective and used randomized trials, however, it was found that no significant evidence proved that an increased rate of completing advance directives and an increased documentation of them led to a reduction in resource utilization among terminally ill patients (Schneiderman, Kronick, Kaplan, Anderson, & Langer, 1992; Teno et al., 1997). In fact, in the study by Teno et al., the average cost of the final hospitalization for those in the intervention group with a written advance directive ($28,017) was greater, but not quite significantly greater, than for those without an advance directive ($24,178).

In terms of hospice care, the argument has been that it saves money by decreasing the amount of more expensive hospital care for the terminally ill (Field & Cassel, 1997). Insofar as actual studies are concerned, however, the situation seems to be much the same as that with advance directives; that is, some retrospective, nonrandomized studies (e.g., Mor & Kidder, 1985; NHO, 1995) have suggested considerable savings. One prospective, randomized trial of hospice care (Kane, Wales, Bernstein, Lebowitz, & Kaplan, 1984) found no evidence of cost savings.

In a critical review of the previous studies, Emanuel (1996) found methodological problems with each of them. For example, the retrospective, nonrandomized studies were subject to a selection bias in the sense that patients who have already chosen to do an advance directive or to enter hospice or palliative care may have preferences for avoiding aggressive treatment. Any savings found with advance directives or hospice care might therefore be attributable to the characteristics of the subjects rather than to the intervention. Similarly, the prospective, advance directive studies selected patients who were very ill at the time of enrollment. Given their condition, such patients might have desired aggressive care in spite of having an advance directive, and conclusions from the study might then not be generalizable.

Emanuel (1996) has further pointed out that it is often difficult to predict how long a particular patient will need to be under hospice care, and the longer the stay in hospice, the less the savings. The primary savings from hospice care (estimated at 25%–40%) occurs in the last month or weeks of life, and most of the savings come from the reduced use of hospitals. For those who stay in a hospice for 6 months or a year, however, the savings can drop to nearly zero percent. This is probably because high-quality hospice or palliative care requires skilled personnel who are not inexpensive. Hospice patients receive care regularly, usually several times a week or daily, depending on their condition, but 3 or 4 months before death, patients receiving conventional care are seen much less frequently.

In any event, Emanuel (1996) concluded that little clear evidence suggests that a windfall of savings could occur from using advance directives, encouraging hospice and palliative care, and generally putting limits on what is considered to be futile treatment. It has been estimated that the most that might be saved by reducing aggressive, life-sustaining care at the end of life might equal approximately 3.3% of the total national health care budget (Emanuel & Emanuel, 1994). Although not insignificant, these savings would hardly be enough to solve the health care problems of the country.

Some modest cost savings may result from the use of advance directives and hospice or palliative care at the end of life. The larger question, however, is whether such savings should be the primary focus of our efforts in this arena. There are many reasons to encourage the completion of advance directives and an entry into hospice or palliative care when a patient is terminally ill. These approaches attempt to respect the individual's wishes; offer compassionate care; promote self-determination and autonomy; protect the patient from overzealous, high-tech rescue efforts; and work at reducing the patient's pain and suffering. If some secondary economic advantage can be achieved as well, that would be a benefit to the healthcare system, but it would seem that our expectations and efforts in this regard should be, at best, restrained.

CONCLUSION

As noted in the preceding sections of this chapter, the increasing ability of medical technology to sustain life, albeit devoid of meaning, and the increasing probability of prolonged dying by degenerative disease seem to have fueled efforts to gain some control and self-determination in the dying process. These efforts have occurred in a culture that generally places great value on individualism and autonomy. The predominant U.S. culture, however, has also been characterized as *youth oriented* and *death denying*. Such characterizations are primarily based on observations of popular culture and, as noted by Field and Cassel (1997), research on this particular issue has been very limited. Moreover, in a pluralistic society such statements run the risk of oversimplification. Yet given a history marked by opportunity and optimism, the Institute of Medicine's Committee on Care at the End of Life (Field & Cassel, 1997) has concluded that the general American unwillingness to accept limits and the tendency to see aging and death as something that research and technology might eliminate have been factors in the approach to end-of-life care in the United States.

As the late historian Arnold Toynbee said, "Death is un-American, an affront to every citizen's right to life, liberty, and the pursuit of happiness" (Callahan, 1995, p. 226). In this regard, the people of the United States are seen not so much as death denying as convinced that if we muster our considerable resources, we can always find ways to overcome disease and prolong active and healthy life. It is this faith in the power of empirical science and technology that can contribute to conflict and disagreement with medical staff who may be struggling with the apparent futility of continued treatment, a topic that will be discussed further in chapter 5. Prior to such discussions, however, it is crucial to have an understanding of the ethical principles and legal issues that guide end-of-life decision making, and these are presented in the next chapter.

APPENDIX: RECENT EFFORTS AT IMPROVED ASSESSMENTS OF QUALITY OF LIFE

Constructing an acceptable quality of life assessment instrument is a formidable task. Cohen and Mount (1992) have noted that most existing quality of life instruments contain items that are inappropriate for a terminally ill, palliative care population. Thus, items that ask about plans for travel, retirement, and long life (see, for example, Ferrans & Powers, 1985) hardly seem relevant or discriminating. Moreover, given the rapid shifts in clinical status and the deficits in memory that many of these patients experience, asking them to rate how they have felt over the past 1–2 weeks may not provide a very accurate assessment. Asking about a single day might also introduce a bias related to temporary shifts in health status, so they have argued that ratings for the past 2 or 3 days may be more appropriate. Because terminally ill patients are generally in poor physical condition, often a need to adapt the method of assessment also exists. Cohen and Mount (1992) have suggested that questionnaires should lend themselves to verbal administration. Those who are very sick may have difficulty grasping the concept of visually presented scales, or they may have difficulty concentrating on items that have multiple options.

Cohen, et al. (1995), the authors of the McGill Quality of Life Questionnaire (MQOL), based their assessment instrument on the thesis of Viktor Frankl (1963) that a sense of quality in life depends on the perception of personal meaning in life. They defined *quality of life* as having a sense of "subjective well-being" (Cohen et al., 1996, p. 576) that, in their framework, would seem to imply a continuing sense or belief that one's life has purpose and value (Cohen & Mount, 1992). In addition to having an articulated conceptual base, the MQOL has a multidimensional structure and assesses for physical symptoms, physical well-being, psychological symptoms, existential well-being, and social support. It allows the patient to specify and rate the particular physical symptoms that are most troublesome to him or her. Ratings in all domains reflect positive and negative contributions to quality of life. Its psychometric properties, including internal consistency, construct validity, and convergent and divergent validity, have been studied and published (Cohen et al., 1995, 1996, 1997). Cohen et al. (1996) have correctly claimed that it meets many of the criteria for quality of life instruments outlined by Gill and Feinstein (1994) in their critical review of this topic. At this point, the MQOL does not allow for a rating of the importance of each item as a contributor to the individual's overall quality of life. It has also been tested primarily on patients with cancer, and so the extent to which its use can be applied to patients with other diagnoses is limited.

Byock and Merriman (1998) have noted that the MQOL was designed for patients in all phases of an illness, including those who may still be curable. They felt a need to develop an instrument that focused more specifically on the terminal phase of illness. They also wanted to have a means of weighing the various measured dimensions according to their importance to the patient, something that, as previously noted, was lacking in the MQOL. The Missoula-VITAS Quality of Life Index (MVQOLI) was constructed with these ends in mind.

The definition of quality of life that the MVQOLI purports to measure has been presented as follows:

> QOL in the context of advanced, progressive, incurable illness is defined as the subjective experience of an individual living with the interpersonal, psychological, and existential or spiritual challenges that accompany the process of physical and functional decline and the knowledge of impending demise. (pp. 233–234)

It is a definition that builds upon a model of lifelong human development that sees the possibility of personal growth even in life's terminal phase (Byock, 1996). Like the MQOL, the MVQOLI also has a multidimensional structure. It is meant to assess for physical symptoms, functional status, interpersonal relationships, subjective well-being, and transcendent meaning and purpose. It does not allow for patient input about symptoms that are particularly problematic for them, but it was developed with information derived from interviews with patients and their families. The study by Byock and Merriman (1998) has reported on the instrument's internal consistency, construct validity, and convergent and divergent validity. The index likewise seems to meet many of the criteria for the assessment of quality of life as they have been put forth by Gill and Feinstein (1994). It is limited in generalizability by the fact that it has only been tested with a population of cancer patients who were predominantly Caucasian and enrolled in hospice programs.

Cohen et al. (1997) have cautioned that scores on any questionnaire or index can never replace the richness of the face-to-face conversation between the dying patient and his or her caregiver. Instruments like the MQOL and the MVQOLI are intended as aids in the evaluation of quality of life. At times, completing them may not only provide a type of measure but may also facilitate the discussion of matters that were previously difficult to broach.

The developers of both the MQOL and the MVQOLI have reported that their instruments are limited by yet another factor, that is, the majority of the terminally ill patients whom they hoped to assess could not complete the task. Cohen et al. (1997), who worked with patients on palliative care services, found that 59% of the patients were ineligible because of weakness or poor mental status. Byock and Merriman (1998), who worked with hospice patients, found that 55% were unable to complete the questionnaire because of an inability to communicate, dementia, or emotional symptoms that might be exacerbated by attempting to do so. Obviously, a sizeable number of terminally ill patients cannot participate in determining their quality of life, yet should clearly not be ignored. As a result, there will also continue to be a place for well-constructed, more objectively oriented measures of quality of life, such as the Support Team Assessment Schedule (Higginson & McCarthy, 1993), which can offer some assistance to caregivers who struggle to understand the patient's quality of life.

2

ETHICAL AND LEGAL ISSUES
IN END-OF-LIFE DECISIONS

No right is held more sacred, or is more carefully guarded by the common law, than the right of every individual to the possession and control of his own person, free from all restraint or interference of others, unless by clear and unquestionable authority of law.

—U.S. Supreme Court
Union Pacific Railway Co. v. Botsford, 141 U.S. 250 (1891)

Given the profound nature of decisions to prolong or not to prolong life, people who are terminally ill, and those family and friends who are involved with them, struggle with complex questions about what is the *right* or ethical thing to do, as well as with questions about what is permitted under the law. The professional staff and the institutions who care for patients with terminal illnesses also struggle with these difficult questions, as does our society more generally. The questions, of course, have always been there, but it is only with the relatively recent developments in medicine and medical technology (as noted in chapter 1) that these questions have been asked by a larger number of people and have therefore come to national attention. The answers are seldom easy, and many points of ethics and law remain unsettled.

As Battin (1994) pointed out, the tensions associated with end-of-life decisions are typically intensified because these decisions are seldom discussed in advance, and they are often made late, or at the eleventh hour, so to speak. Because these decisions have to do with such a profound event for the individual, a natural inclination is to postpone making them. Thus, even though advance care planning through the completion of *advance directives* or the designation of a health care proxy is now encouraged, only a minority of patients have attended to such matters. Health care staff and families are therefore often faced with the need to determine the wishes of a patient who is debilitated and in a fluctuating state of awareness. Given such circumstances, it is important to have a good grounding in the ethical and legal bases for end-of-life decision making.

In this chapter, we initially discuss the ethical principles pertinent to end-of-life decisions. We also examine the legal bases for such decisions, including the legal theory of informed consent; its most debated element, competency or decision-making capacity; and how it may be assessed. The chapter is intended to provide guidelines for thinking about and making decisions about the issues presented in subsequent chapters of this book.

THE ETHICAL PRINCIPLES THAT GUIDE END-OF-LIFE DECISION MAKING AND THEIR APPLICATION

Ethicists who have examined end-of-life issues have put forth several principles to guide the life or death decision-making process. Autonomy, beneficence, mercy, nonmaleficence, and justice are principles that are not unique to issues in the final phase of life, but they are nonetheless frequently cited in that context. As these principles are discussed here, it needs to be emphasized again that they have been derived from our dominant European American tradition, and they may be viewed quite differently by those from different cultural groups within our society (Werth, Blevins, Toussaint, & Durham, 2002).

Ethical Decision-Making Models

Even within the context of the predominant culture, some controversy surrounds the application of these principles, or whether to apply them at all, when arriving at ethical decisions. In this regard, Beauchamp and Childress (2001) articulated three influential models for justifying ethical judgments. The first is the so-called top-down or deductive model in which one starts with an ethical principle or principles and applies them to a particular case. In this model, absolute principles are given priority over the complexities of individual cases. Such an approach often leads to the position that there can be only one correct account of the ethics of the situation and it is based on the principles that have been applied.

The second decision-making model is the so-called bottom-up or inductive model in which the reasoning moves from particular cases to general statements or positions. This model de-emphasizes reasoning from principles, because principles are seen as derivatives of actual case experiences. The bottom-up model has been criticized for its failure to provide a stable ethical framework and its difficulty in preventing prejudicial conclusions and conventions.

The third model is an integrated one in which the extremes of the other two models are eschewed and it is maintained that "principles need to be made specific for cases, and case analysis needs illumination from general principles" (Beauchamp & Childress, 2001, p. 397). In effect, the model suggests an assimilation and accommodation process in which clinicians are guided by principles but open to adjustment based on particular cases and circumstances.

It is this third model that will be used to frame the approach favored in this book. The specific principles mentioned earlier are defined in the following paragraphs. Given the preferred approach to arriving at ethical decisions , it should be clear that these principles are not intended to be applied in an inflexible or absolute fashion.

The Principle of Autonomy

In our society, and especially in the dominant cultural group, the ethical principle of autonomy, as noted earlier, is highly valued and has been viewed by many as the very foundation for decisions that hasten death or prolong life (Wachter & Lo, 1993). The principle has been stated as follows:

> One ought to respect a competent person's choices, where one can do so without undue cost to oneself, where to do so will not violate other moral obligations, and where these choices do not threaten harm to other persons or parties. (Battin, 1994, p. 107)

When applied to end-of-life decision making, this principle asserts that competent individuals should have the right to make their own decisions about such things as accepting or refusing medical treatment, whether that means life or death for them, provided that it is a thoughtful choice and does not create harm for others. Furthermore, autonomy should not be restricted by the limitations that others establish through their own personal values or standards (Fulbrook, 1994).

Opposing concerns exist about the application of the principle of autonomy. On the one hand, some have taken issue with the weight given to autonomy in American bioethics. As Beauchamp and Childress (2001) pointed out, some feel that strong proponents of self-determination may unintentionally attempt to force patients to make choices that they would just as soon not make. Many patients may want to be informed about their illness, but might prefer to leave health care decisions to the medical staff or to the family. It is clearly important to listen to patients' wishes in this regard and to try to take into account their particular value systems.

On the other hand, autonomy (or self-governance) is often contrasted with *paternalism* in which another person interferes with or controls another's choices in the interests of what they perceive as that person's *own good* or welfare. Some paternalistic acts, such as preventing someone who is in a delirium from leaving an emergency room (ER), are clearly beneficent because the individual has been rendered temporarily incapacitated from making his or her own competent choices and would be at serious risk. Paternalistically overriding a mentally clear and competent patient's choice to leave an ER without being treated for a condition such as hypertension, however, would be incompatible with the principle of autonomy.

In the realm of health care, it is typically those with expert knowledge who may be inclined to act paternalistically and ignore a competent patient's choices. These situations tend to arise because of the medical staff's authoritative position and the patient's dependent condition (Beauchamp & Childress, 2001). Regarding a patient who is terminally ill yet competent, those who would interfere with the patient's autonomous choice must consider to what extent they are acting on their own values, rather than on those of the individual in question. They must also consider the cost of intervening, which might mean continued and unwanted suffering (Battin, 1994). In the U.S. health care system, autonomous choice is widely viewed as a patient's right if he or she chooses to exercise it. The obligation of the health care staff is to respect autonomous choice and, in addition, to foster it appropriately (i.e., to facilitate it as a right, but not to insist on it as a duty).

The Principle of Beneficence

Beneficence, as noted earlier, is an action intended to benefit others. It constitutes the fundamental purpose and rationale for medicine and the health care professions in general. A principle of beneficence in health care refers to a moral obligation to act for the benefit of others (Beauchamp & Childress, 2001). In health care, the obligation of beneficent treatment derives from the fiduciary relationship between the patient and the treatment provider. When a treatment provider enters into an explicit or implicit contract to provide services to a patient, a commitment and a subsequent obligation are made to attempt to meet the health needs of the patient and to promote his or her well-being.

Given the centrality of beneficence to the functioning of physicians and health care staff, and the value placed on autonomous choice for patients in our society, it should come as no surprise that it is not infrequent that conflicts arise over which principle, beneficence or autonomy, applies and should have priority (refer to the previous discussion of paternalism). In this regard, Beauchamp and Childress (2001) pointed out that it is entirely possible, and perhaps best, not to view these principles as competing. Rather, their view is that beneficence provides the primary goal of health care, while autonomy (and other ethical principles) places moral limits on the professional's efforts to pursue this goal. In this framework, no principle in bioethics is preeminent over another, but, in effect, the patient needs to listen to and understand the goals of the physician or health care team, while the team must respect the autonomous choices of the competent patient. Moreover, one might argue that a beneficent perspective on the part of the medical staff would include the patient's choices as part of what determines the most comprehensive benefit for him or her.

The Principle of Mercy

The principle of mercy, as used here, has to do with mercy in regard to medical conditions. It should be distinguished from judicial mercy as in the granting of a pardon. Some bioethicists have subsumed mercy under a broadly defined principle of beneficence (Beauchamp & Childress, 2001), while others have treated it separately because of its particular relevance in some end-of-life decisions (Battin, 1994). The latter position has been adopted in this book and the following definition of the principle of mercy will be used:

> Where possible, one ought to relieve the pain or suffering of another person, when it does not contravene that person's wishes, where one can do so without undue costs to oneself, where one will not violate other moral obligations, where the pain or suffering itself is not necessary for the sufferer's attainment of some overriding good, and where the pain or suffering can be relieved without precluding the sufferer's attainment of some overriding good. (Battin, 1994, p. 101)

Thus, the principle of mercy refers to the duty to relieve or end suffering that is currently occurring. It is invoked as a justification for certain end-of-life decisions that result in hastening death. An example might be the terminally ill patient for whom usual pain management has failed, who is suffering unbearably, and for whom the only relief might come from an increase in medication that could also result in the shortening of a life that is already coming to an end. Provided that the patient, or his or her surrogate, is in agreement, the most merciful act might be to relieve the pain even though death might follow closely. This type of decision is also referred to as invoking the principle of the *double effect* and will be discussed further in chapter 3.

The Principle of Nonmaleficence

The principle of nonmaleficence has roots in the medical directive *primum non nocere* or *first do no harm*. This directive is widely believed to stem from the Hippocratic oath, but its actual origins seem to be more obscure (Beauchamp & Childress, 2001). Nonmalficence cautions the health care provider to refrain from tests and procedures that may inflict suffering when no overriding benefit will occur, such as relief from pain or improvement in the patient's condition. Thus, for example, cardiopulmonary resuscitation (CPR) is a procedure that can be used in response to a cardiac arrest, but it can also result in substantial injury and subsequent physical pain. Its use is justified if a hope for survival exists; however, repeated use of it in the case of a patient who is terminally ill, wishes to die, and has little hope of meaningful or beneficial survival could cause great physical damage while little or nothing would be gained.

Some (e.g., Battin, 1994) have seen nonmalficence as a component of the principle of mercy in that it warns us not to inflict pain and suffering needlessly. Others (e.g., Committee on Bioethics, 1994; Headley, 1991) have seen it as related to the principle of beneficence in that it directs us not to act in ways that would be the opposite of beneficial. In fact, nonmaleficence seems to have features that could be characterized as both merciful and beneficent. For the sake of clarity, it is discussed here as separate but related to both the principles of mercy and beneficence.

The Principle of Justice

According to Beauchamp and Childress (2001), the concept of justice refers to "fair, equitable, and appropriate treatment in light of what is due or owed to persons" (p. 226). Someone who has a *just* claim has a right to, or is owed, something. Someone who has suffered an *injustice* has been denied some benefit that is rightly his or hers or has been given some unfair burden. In the realm of end-of-life care, or health care in general, the concerns with justice that most often arise are typically considered under the rubric of *distributive justice*. Distributive justice is to be distinguished from other forms of justice such as *criminal justice* or *social justice*. It refers to the fair distribution of rights and responsibilities, and, insofar as health care is concerned, it generally refers to the right to a fair distribution of services and resources.

Unfortunately, our society has not reached a consensus on a set of principles or rules that can be used to arrive at distributive justice in health care. As a result, as Beauchamp and Childress (2001) indicated, many parts of the U.S. health care system are unfair. Should health care be given according to equal share, need, some system of merit, the ability to pay, the potential benefit, and so forth? These are questions that have not been answered. Rather, we have left access to health insurance, and consequently access to health care, to be determined by socioeconomic factors. Thus, about 60% of the U.S. population has employer-based health insurance, another 25% has some form of publicly supported health insurance or private insurance, and the remaining 15% (or approximately 44 million people) have no health insurance. Some are denied or can only receive limited insurance coverage because of exclusionary clauses for preexisting conditions that could lead to expensive future claims. These people are thus denied coverage for the very conditions for which they most need medical care.

Another level of difficulty with distributive justice in health care occurs when particular services and resources are scarce, causing an increased competition for them. When an illness is life threatening and a scarce resource can be life saving, decisions about who is treated and who is not can quickly become a question of who will live and who will not. Requests for heart, lung, liver, and kidney transplants are prototypical examples of situations in which demand exceeds resources (i.e., donated organs). In 1972, Congress voted to provide funding for renal dialysis and kidney transplantation for any citizen of the United States with end-stage renal disease (ESRD; Olbrisch, 1996). Such has not been the case for those with end-stage heart or liver disease. Yet even with requests for kidney transplantation, no standardized format or criteria has been determined for who is an appropriate transplant candidate versus who must continue with dialysis. In addition, indications show that decisions have been skewed by social class, income, age, race, and gender (Kutner, 1994; Normand, 1994). It seems clear that we have much to learn and do before we can say that scarce medical resources can be allotted justly and equitably.

The Ethical Decision-Making Process

As indicated at the beginning of this section, the principles mentioned above will not automatically lead us to decisions or conclusions about particular end-of-life situations. They offer guidance on acting to benefit the patient, respecting his or her choices, and treating him or her fairly. In actual cases, however, more than one principle may apply, and these principles may seem to be in conflict with each other. Thus, for example, some of the seminal end-of-life cases like *Quinlan* and *Cruzan* (in which medical staff opposed the family's wishes to discontinue the patient's life-sustaining treatment) have involved apparent conflicts between beneficence and nonmalficence on the one hand and autonomy (as exercised by a surrogate in these cases) on the other. Such conflicts make the need for a process of moral reasoning and judgment apparent.

Again, it is important to keep in mind that no exact guide to action can be established from the framework of these ethical principles. Moreover, it is likely that ambiguity and controversy will always be associated with ethical decision making. If it is found that two or more ethical principles apply to a case but are in conflict, then it is necessary to go through a process of deliberation (such as that suggested for the integrated model of decision making noted earlier). That is, one needs to examine the relative merits and strengths of the arguments for each principle in light of the circumstances of the particular case. If better reasons can be offered for one principle, and no preferable alternative actions are available, then that principle (and the action it implies) will override the other. The process of reaching such a decision involves testing, rejecting, and modifying the available facts and arguments until a considered judgment is reached and can be held with some confidence.

THE LEGAL BASES FOR END-OF-LIFE DECISIONS

In American law, as in American bioethics, the concept and value of individual autonomy have very deep roots. They reverberate through the U.S. Supreme Court statement cited at the beginning of this chapter (p. 27), as well as through the ruling in 1914 attributed to U.S. Supreme Court Justice Benjamin Cardozo that "every human being of adult years of sound mind has a right to determine what shall be done with his [or her] own body" (Nicholson & Matross, 1989, p. 234). Although those in bioethics (e.g., Beauchamp & Childress, 2001) might want to see an integrative approach to the interests of autonomy and the interests of beneficence, in American law, autonomy or self-determination has almost invariably triumphed over interest in promoting the patient's benefit, the exception being those cases in which the patient's judgment is significantly impaired (Grisso & Appelbaum, 1998). It comes as no surprise then that judicial statements such as those just noted have become building blocks in the legal foundation of the doctrine of informed consent/refusal, a doctrine that lies at the heart of end-of-life decision making.

The Law and the Refusal of Life-Sustaining Treatment

It is a curious fact that the legal acceptance of the right to refuse life-sustaining treatment was given great impetus in recent times by the case mentioned in chapter 1, that of Karen Ann Quinlan, a young woman who was clearly unable to consent to or refuse anything (*In re Quinlan*, 1976). In this case, the Supreme Court of New Jersey argued that Karen Ann Quinlan, despite the opposition of her treatment providers, had the right to have the mechanical ventilator that was helping to sustain her life disconnected. Because she was in an irreversible vegetative state and could not personally exercise her right, the court further ruled that her parents could act as surrogates for her and make a substituted judgment on this issue. The fact that the hospital and the medical staff had felt compelled to continue Ms. Quinlan's existence, although it seemed devoid of meaning to her family, set off alarms about whether individuals could have any control over the process of their own dying. Given that the court accepted Ms. Quinlan's parents as representatives of her interests, the decision in this case also validated what is now an accepted practice in many jurisdictions, that is, asking family members to act as surrogate decision makers for patients who are incompetent and critically ill.

In another prominent and related case (*Cruzan v. Director, Missouri Department of Health*, 1990), the Supreme Court recognized a *liberty interest* (under the Fourteenth Amendment) in refusing unwanted medical treatment, including artificially administered nutrition and hydration. The young woman in this case, Nancy Beth Cruzan, was also in a persistent vegetative state and unable to make her own health care decisions following a car accident. The medical staff felt that she had no hope of recovery. Based on statements she had made prior to the accident, her parents maintained that she would not want to live in her condition. They sought to have the feeding tube that sustained her life removed. This request was eventually granted by a state court and she died 12 days later.

According to Luce and Alpers (2001), the right of a competent patient to refuse life-sustaining treatment was more directly established in two cases. First, in *Bartling v. Superior Court* (1984), a California Court of Appeal held that a patient could be removed from a mechanical ventilator at his request and over the objections of his physician and his hospital. Second, in *Bouvia v. Superior Court* (1986), another California Court of Appeal held that a conscious and competent hospitalized patient who was in severe and intractable pain could refuse nutrition and hydration with the understanding that it would hasten her death.

In the Cruzan case, the Supreme Court held that the state of Missouri could impose procedural safeguards and require that there be *clear and convincing evidence* that the refusal of life-sustaining treatment would be what an incompetent individual would have wanted for him- or herself. Casual statements to family or friends prior to becoming incompetent were not seen as adequate (Burke, 1996). The ruling also raised questions about the practice of simply respecting family decision making on behalf of the incompetent patient. Nancy Beth Cruzan's parents were eventually able to bring forth new witnesses who had had specific discussions with their daughter prior to her accident about not wanting to be kept alive in a state of permanent unconsciousness. As noted earlier, the state court then authorized the removal of artificial nutrition and hydration.

Related to its ruling in this case, the Supreme Court advocated the use of advance directives to protect the autonomy of individuals. An advance directive is a declaration, while the individual is still competent, about what treatment they would or would not want if they lost their decision-making capacity. Several states (e.g., California and North Carolina) had previously passed so-called *living will* or *natural death* statutes in which they established the right of their citizens to complete such directives. This right was recognized by the Supreme Court in the Cruzan case.

Prompted in part by the Cruzan case (which had been moving through the state of Missouri's court system in the 1980s), Senator John Danforth of Missouri sponsored the Patient Self-Determination Act (PSDA) and the U.S. Congress enacted it on December 1, 1991 (Prendergast, 2001). The

PSDA was an attempt to encourage advance care planning through the more extensive use of advance directives. This legislation applied to all health care facilities, including hospitals, nursing homes, hospices, managed care organizations, and home health care agencies that participate in Medicare or Medicaid and receive federal funds. The PSDA required these institutions to provide written information to patients about their rights to accept or refuse medical treatment and to complete advance directives. The goal of this statute was both to encourage the use of advance directives and to prompt health care institutions to honor these documents (Wolf et al., 1991). Although difficulties arose with the use of advance directives, the enactment of this legislation put the federal government and the nation on record as sanctioning responsible decisions by terminally ill patients to refuse life-sustaining treatments that might only prolong the dying process.

The Law and Decisions That May Hasten Death

In two significant cases (*Washington v. Glucksberg*, 1997; *Vacco v. Quill*, 1997), the Supreme Court found no constitutional right to physician-assisted suicide. They ruled that the states of Washington and New York could, in fact, prohibit assisted suicide, but they also allowed that individual states, if they wished, could legalize the practice. The state of Oregon has done so.

The cases of *Glucksberg* and *Vacco* have been introduced here not to prompt a discussion of assisted suicide, but because it is in these cases that the court also addressed the right to be free from unnecessary pain during the dying process (Luce & Alpers, 2001). In effect, the court accepted the principle of double effect and, with it, drew a distinction between assisted suicide and what was referred to as palliative care. According to the principle of double effect, one can perform an act that has a foreseen bad effect (e.g., death) and still be judged in a morally favorable light as long as one does not intend the bad effect and only intends the good one (e.g., relief from otherwise intractable pain). Many questions have been raised about this principle as an ethical guide (see chapter 3), but under it, the court has justified acts such as giving sedatives and analgesics that lead to the relief of pain while also possibly hastening death in terminally ill patients. In these cases, the bad effect of death may be foreseen, but it must not be the physician's intent.

In situations where medication is given to relieve pain or where life support is withdrawn and medication is given to provide comfort and reduce suffering, Luce and Alpers (2001) cautioned that the palliative measures used should be dictated by objective signs of patient distress whenever possible. Although wide variations can take place in the amount of pain medication needed to provide relief, the physician should be careful that sedatives and analgesics are given in doses that target pain relief, but not in doses that would suggest that they are being given primarily to cause death. Likewise, neuromuscular blocking agents that prevent spontaneous breathing should not be introduced when a ventilator is withdrawn because they do not con-tribute to comfort and suggest an intention to bring about death. Patients in such circumstances can usually be kept comfortable with small doses of nar-cotics and benzodiazepines.

The Supreme Court's adoption of the principle of double effect has been interpreted as extending to approval for the practice of terminal sedation (Luce & Alpers, 2001). In terminal sedation, the terminally ill patient is ren-dered comatose with medication and has other treatments withdrawn, including nutrition and hydration. This interpretation is based on opinions in the cases of *Glucksberg* and *Vacco* by at least two justices who wrote of the need, in some instances, for sedation to the point of unconsciousness to relieve pain, even if to do so would hasten death (Burt, 1997). An argument against permitting terminal sedation has been that the intent of withdraw-ing life-sustaining treatment in these cases is not to relieve pain and suffer-ing, but to bring about death (Orentlicher, 1997). The counterargument, however, has been that the patient or his or her surrogate may make an informed decision to have unwanted treatment (such as artificial nutrition and hydration) withdrawn while accepting sedation to the point of uncon-sciousness to eliminate suffering while dying.

Essential Elements of the Legal Doctrine of Informed Consent

Although physicians generally do not treat people without their con-sent, Grisso and Appelbaum (1998) pointed out that it was not until the mid-20th century that the courts began to seriously question the extent to which patients' interests were being protected under an informal system based on trust and the assumption of benevolent paternalism. Increasingly, they focused on the patient's right to make autonomous decisions about things that affected him or her so intimately as health care, especially health care that had a bearing on the time and conditions of dying. One of the seminal cases in the development of the doctrine of informed consent was the case of *Natanson v. Kline* (1960) in which the Kansas Supreme Court stated in gen-eral terms what information a physician should provide for patients prior to asking for their consent to treatment. This information included the nature and purpose of the proposed treatment, its potential benefits and risks, any alternative treatments, and their potential benefits and risks (Grisso & Appelbaum, 1998). Information, however, is only one of three elements in modern-day informed consent.

An informed consent procedure ensures patients' rights to be edu-cated adequately about the nature and consequences of any proposed med-ical treatment so that they can make an informed decision about whether they want to accept or refuse the treatment (Simon, 1994). The three major components of informed consent are information, voluntariness, and competency.

As just noted, the first component supports the patient's right to have sufficient *information* to be able to make a reasoned decision about the treatment. Standards for what defines a legally sufficient disclosure can vary from state to state. Initially, the standard most commonly applied was measured from the professional's standpoint or "what a reasonable physician would disclose under the circumstances or the customary disclosure practices of physicians in a particular community" (Simon, 1994, p. 1306). Grisso and Appelbaum (1998) pointed out, however, that this professional standard eventually came to be viewed by the courts as contrary to the motivation behind the development of informed consent law. Informed consent law has in part been motivated by the perception that physicians were not sharing enough information with patients to allow them to make meaningful choices. Thus, over time, the courts have shifted toward a patient-oriented standard that focuses on information that would *materially affect* a patient's decision, or "information that a reasonable person in the patient's position would want to know in order to make a reasonably informed decision" (Simon, 1994, p. 1306) about the risks and benefits of accepting or refusing the various treatment options.

The next component of informed consent is *voluntariness*. The medical staff must attempt to insure that the circumstances surrounding the consent process are free of coercion, threats, or fraud, and the patient should not be experiencing duress that affects his or her decision-making ability (Simon, 1994). Even though the staff may be convinced of the benefits of treatment, threats such as the possibility of withdrawing from the patient's care unless the patient agrees to a specific plan of treatment are unacceptable. This, of course, does not mean that there may not be circumstances when a patient's complete refusal to cooperate makes treatment futile. In such cases, withdrawal of care may be possible if, for example, the option of alternative care is available to the patient (Grisso & Appelbaum, 1998). The precautions about avoiding coercive practices should also not be taken as a deterrent to recommending what the medical staff believes to be the best course of treatment. Clearly, one of the services of a clinician is to use his or her expertise to help the patient distinguish which options seem most viable under the given circumstances.

Competency, the third element of informed consent, has been the component most discussed and debated in the literature. It implies that one has the basic cognitive and functional capacities to participate in the decision-making process. Technically speaking, *competence* is a legal term, and in our legal system an individual is considered competent to make his or her own decisions, unless declared otherwise by a duly appointed court of law (Mishkin, 1989). As Grisso and Appelbaum (1998) pointed out, most authors in this field have distinguished between the assessments of decision-making capacities, which clinicians can do, and the determinations of competence or incompetence, which are based on such assessments but are made by the courts. In actual practice, the terms competent and incompetent seem to be used freely, perhaps too freely, in clinical situations. Four standards for competence have been used regularly in court decisions (Grisso & Appelbaum, 1995a) but in ambiguous and inconsistent ways. These standards and the complex issues that surround them are discussed in greater detail in the next section.

Although it is legally important to obtain an informed consent before providing treatment, and failure to do so can make one liable for any harm that may result, this requirement has four exceptions. The first exception can occur in emergency situations when immediate treatment is necessary and consent cannot be obtained because the patient is unable to provide it (e.g., the patient is in a coma) or time constraints prevent obtaining it. The potential progression of events must be serious and imminent, and the emergency must be determined by the patient's condition and not the environmental or surrounding situation, such as a lack of resources (Simon, 1994).

A second exception to informed consent occurs when a patient has been declared legally incompetent to make treatment decisions. When this occurs, a substitute decision maker needs to be identified who will try to make decisions as the patient would if competent. Such substituted judgment works best if the patient had a known set of values or was known to act in consistent ways in regard to health care.

A third condition in which treatment providers are exempt from obtaining informed consent occurs when a patient waives his or her right to be fully informed. To waive his or her right, a patient must be fully aware of the nature of the request, be competent enough to make this decision, and be making it voluntarily.

The fourth exception to informed consent is known as *therapeutic privilege*. It is rarely invoked, but is applicable when it has been determined that full disclosure about the treatment options and the associated risks might have a negative impact on the patient (Simon, 1994). The necessary conditions for this exception to be applied are vague, and as the emphasis on patient autonomy expands in our society, fewer justifiable instances may occur when this more paternalistic action can be condoned.

As noted above, when a patient no longer has the capacity to give an informed consent or refusal, a surrogate decision maker needs to be appointed. Clinicians should understand, however, that identifying a substitute decision maker is not necessarily an easy way to achieve direction in a case. Clearly, there are patients who, although incapable of autonomous decision making, can still refuse to cooperate with or assent to a treatment that their surrogate believes they would want were they in a more capable state of mind. Thus, some incompetent patients can be so actively or passively resistant that they may seriously compromise the treatment or procedure itself or any crucial aftercare such as compliance with medications or physical therapy. In these situations, the surrogate must carefully consider the patient's known values and directives (or best interests as the case may be) in relation to the likelihood of successful treatment and the suffering that may ensue when efforts are made to treat the patient against his or her will.

EVALUATING DECISION-MAKING CAPACITY AND DETERMINING COMPETENCY

Given the fact that terminally ill patients often have conditions that can seriously effect their mental capacities, and given the gravity of the decisions that must be made, it is very important that those clinicians who work with them have an understanding of how they might attempt to evaluate decision-making capacity and determine the patient's ability to participate in decisions about accepting or refusing treatment. Auerbach and Banja (1993) have pointed out that although mental health professionals are routinely involved in evaluations that provide a basis for legal decisions about competency, most of them are poorly versed in the significant issues related to this process.

Take, for example, the case of Mr. G.[1] Mr. G was a 62-year-old, divorced, Caucasian male who was admitted to a cardiac care unit (CCU) with chest pain and a history of heart attacks. Cardiac catheterization revealed severe three-vessel coronary artery disease that the surgical team felt required immediate bypass surgery, lest his arteries become completely occluded. The patient had a psychiatric history in which, 35 years ago, he had been diagnosed as having paranoid schizophrenia, but his diagnosis was subsequently changed to bipolar disorder. The patient seemed somewhat overwhelmed by this new information about his cardiac condition and he refused to consent to the bypass surgery. He said that he wanted a second opinion, and when pressed to accept the surgery, he asked to leave the hospital against medical advice. A mental health consultation was requested to assess the patient's capacity to refuse treatment.

The mental health consultant examined the patient and found that he was not currently exhibiting either acute psychotic symptoms or an acute mood disorder. The patient was also found to be free from any suicidal ideation. He was, however, distrustful of the surgical staff's opinion about his condition. The patient explained that he had been misdiagnosed with paranoid schizophrenia in the past, and that he had been treated with medications, one of which gave him the very unpleasant side effect of contractions in his neck while another caused sexual dysfunction. Since that time, he had been wary of diagnoses and treatment recommendations. In spite of this explanation, the consultant, who was understandably worried that the patient could die in the near future if he refused the bypass, concluded that

---

[1] The case of Mr. G is based on an actual case, but certain aspects of the case have been changed to ensure confidentiality.

he had an underlying psychotic thought process that impaired his judgment and that he did not have the decision-making capacity to refuse treatment.

The CCU staff disagreed with this opinion and felt very uncomfortable about the possibility of doing such invasive surgery against the patient's will. They requested a consultation from the hospital's Ethics Advisory Committee (EAC). A subcommittee of the EAC (that included a mental health staff member) evaluated the patient and came to the conclusion that, in their opinion, he met the criteria for decision-making capacity. They discussed the situation with the mental health consultant and the CCU staff, and the subcommittee recommended that the patient be told that he was free to accept or refuse treatment, but that the staff wanted to discuss his condition and the potential consequences of refusing treatment further with him. After the discussion, and understanding that the treatment was not being forced on him, the patient consented to the bypass surgery, which had a very successful outcome.

Until recent times, mental illness and mental retardation were often thought to imply a lack of decision-making capacity. Moreover, people were thought to be either universally competent or universally incompetent; that is, competency was considered an all-or-none affair. As Kleespies and Mori (1998) pointed out, however, court decisions and legislation have moved competency proceedings in the direction of an approach that emphasizes functional abilities with regard to discrete domains of behavior (e.g., competence to refuse treatment or competence to stand trial), rather than attempting to say that a person is either competent or incompetent for all functions.

Given that the terms competence and incompetence have specific legal meanings, psychologists and other mental health practitioners need to observe some caution about how they express themselves in this regard. The author believes that it is best to express opinions about the functional abilities of an individual and to leave the determination of competence or incompetence to either the courts or to an approved institutional process. For those in mental health, the language of competency is best replaced by the language of decision-making capacity (Auerbach & Banja, 1993). Having said this, however, it is important to note that Grisso and Appelbaum (1998) maintained that clinicians might do well if they attempted to mimic the process that would be used in court to determine competence or incompetence. Because some cases could proceed to the court for adjudication, it will be important to demonstrate that, in effect, the court's criteria were applied. The standards or criteria that follow are essentially those that have evolved through the legal process.

Standards or Criteria for Competency

Over the past 25 years, a concerted effort has been made to define the so-called tests or criteria for competency to consent to or refuse treatment (Kleespies & Mori, 1998). Initially, some hope existed that the field might agree on a single acceptable criterion. In the words of Roth, Meisel, and Lidz

(1977), however, this quest was eventually abandoned as "a search for a Holy Grail" (p. 283). Because judgments of competence or incompetence reflect not only medical and legal issues but also complex psychosocial issues as well as societal mores, traditions, and biases, it was recognized that there could be no single criterion.

Two other issues seem to have been worked through and discarded. First, Roth et al. (1977) originally suggested five tests for competency, one of which was referred to as the *reasonable outcome of choice*. This proposed criterion was questioned as contrary to the value that our society places on personal autonomy. It entailed making a decision that was roughly equivalent to a decision that a reasonable person in similar circumstances would make. Frequently, however, the decision of a reasonable person was defined as that of the physician or of the treatment staff. The criterion was rejected as biased in favor of accepting treatment.

Second, in an effort to resolve the complicated issue of standards of competency for treatment decisions that were associated with widely varying medical conditions, Drane (1984) proposed a sliding standard: "The more dangerous the medical decision, the more stringent the standards of competency" (p. 926). This approach was seriously criticized by Sullivan and Youngner (1994) who objected to the fact that Drane's proposal linked the criteria to outcome. They argued that this linkage would erode the independence of the competence determination from the treatment decision in question. In other words, a potential refusal of treatment, even though it might mean that the patient died, should not be the basis for altering the criteria for competence and certainly should not be the basis for a determination of incompetence. As McCrary and Walman (1990) indicated, competency evaluation should be based on an assessment of the patient's processes of understanding and reasoning, not on the content of his or her decision. To this criticism, Venesy (1994) added that a sliding standard would make it more likely that a patient's views could be outweighed by a physician's views in that the physician has control over shifts in what standard would be applied.

Grisso and Appelbaum (1995a) reported that four standards or criteria for competency were most frequently found in case law. They were (a) the ability to express a choice, (b) the ability to understand information relevant to the decision about treatment, (c) the ability to appreciate the significance of the information disclosed for one's own illness and possible treatment, and (d) the ability to reason with relevant information so as to engage in a logical process of weighing treatment options. Their investigations focused on these four criteria in an effort to define which of them might prove useful as tests of competency.

Although these standards were cited in case law, it has never been settled, either clinically or legally, as to whether one is to accept and apply one standard, all four standards, or some combination of two or three. There is little doubt that if one standard or set of standards is applied and is either more or less demanding than the others, it can affect patients' autonomy in decision making. Overly demanding criteria would have the effect of ruling out people who should perhaps be allowed to make their own end-of-life decisions, while criteria that demand too little might fail to protect people who are incapacitated and at risk of making poor judgments (Grisso & Appelbaum, 1995a).

The first standard (i.e., the ability to express a choice) was seen by Kleespies and Mori (1998, p. 155) as a "sine qua non" and has been referred to by Grisso and Appelbaum (1998) as a *threshold* issue. Thus, if patients are incapable of making their wishes known or of making a choice, they can make no decision even if, by some chance, the other criteria of understanding, appreciation, and rationality could be assessed. Typically, however, if a patient cannot express a choice, assessing the other functional abilities is not necessary. The exception to this rule occurs when the inability to express a choice is transient, as can happen, for example, in mild to moderate states of dementia. In these instances, the clinician needs to assess decision-making capacity during the patient's more lucid periods.

The other question, of course, is whether the ability to express a choice is adequate in and of itself as a criterion for competency. As Grisso and Appelbaum (1998) pointed out, this would set a very low threshold. Although someone who is incapable of understanding the relevant information, of appreciating the implications of a particular illness for him- or herself, and of thinking rationally about his or her condition might still be able to express a choice, it would seem to be a choice that runs counter to the entire notion of informed consent or refusal.

It seems logical to regard the ability to express a choice as a necessary but not a sufficient criterion for competency. It must be taken in conjunction with one or more of the other three criteria. The second criterion, that the patient be able to understand information relevant to the decision about treatment, also seems like a basic requirement in any meaningful informed consent. If the patient is incapable of a basic understanding of what is being proposed, it seems difficult to maintain that the patient can be truly informed. It should come as no surprise that understanding is the criterion most frequently referred to by the courts, the legislatures, and ethicists when decision-making capacity is discussed. According to Grisso and Appelbaum (1992), this criterion refers to the patient's capacity to comprehend the meaning and intent of the following information: (a) the nature of the disorder or injury, (b) the nature of the recommended treatment, (c) the likely benefits of the treatment, (d) the likely risks and discomforts of the treatment, and (e) any alternative treatments and their relative risks and benefits.

The third standard or criterion listed earlier goes beyond the simple understanding of information and requires an ability to appreciate the significance of the information for one's own illness and possible treatment. Thus, one can understand that death is a likely consequence if someone with ESRD refuses dialysis, yet not believe that one has ESRD. Appelbaum and

Grisso (1992) noted that legal incompetence under this standard means that one fails to recognize that one has a particular illness or fails to accept the relevance of an appropriate treatment for one's condition. Beyond this, however, this standard also requires that such failures of recognition stem from cognitive deficits or emotional states in which the patient's beliefs about his or her illness or treatment are irrational, delusional, and not reality based. If a patient rigidly denies symptoms to avoid the emotional pain related to his or her condition, it could be considered indicative of a *defense-based* denial or lack of appreciation. Likewise, if a patient has a neurological impairment that leads to a denial of an illness, it would be considered indicative of an *organic-based* lack of appreciation.

On the other hand, Appelbaum and Grisso (1992) cautioned that there can also be *reality-based* and *value-based* disavowals of the efficacy of treatment or the basis of a disease. These disavowals occur when, for example, a patient has had personal experience with many past efforts at treatment that have failed and he or she has little basis on which to believe that a new treatment effort will have any greater success. Disavowals can also occur when a patient's religious or cultural beliefs are in conflict with a proposed medical intervention. Disavowals such as these could hardly be considered as consistent with a determination of incompetence.

The fourth criterion is that the patient shows the ability to reason with relevant information so as to engage in a logical process of weighing treatment options. According to Grisso and Appelbaum (1993), this refers to the quality of the patient's mental operations, not to the quality or reasonableness of his or her actual choice. It is distinct from understanding, for example, insofar as one can engage in a logical thinking process, even though information is misunderstood, or engage in illogical thinking with accurately understood information. Grisso and Appelbaum (1993; 1998) suggested that a wide range of cognitive abilities contributes to the rational processing of information during decision making (e.g., attention, memory, abstract thinking, and problem solving). After a review of the cognitive theories of decision making and problem solving, they proposed the following elements as most relevant to a determination of a rational thought process in decision making.

First, evidence must show that the individual can stay focused on the problem of selecting a treatment. Second, the person must demonstrate an ability to take into account the range of available options, or at least consider more than a single alternative, while processing the decision. Third, the decision maker must demonstrate an ability to generate future, practical consequences of the different possible treatment choices for his or her life. Fourth, the patient must be able to realize the likelihood that particular consequences might occur. Fifth, the individual must weigh the desirability of the various consequences given his or her values. Finally, the patient must show evidence of deliberating and comparing the relevant consequences or potential outcomes and their likelihood and desirability.

Grisso and Appelbaum (1995a) studied two related questions pertinent to the use of the three standards: understanding, appreciation, and rational thinking. The first question is whether patients impaired on one standard tended to be impaired on the other two standards as well. If so, it might indicate that the three criteria are not distinct and are measuring the same essential ability. The second question is whether a hierarchy of rigorousness exists among these three criteria, such that one or the other is more difficult to meet. If so, it might assist in gauging the difficulty of meeting a particular standard or combination of standards.

Using data from a large, multisite controlled study of decision-making capacities, Grisso and Appelbaum assessed three groups of patients (schizophrenic patients, depressive patients, and patients with ischemic heart disease) with three instruments developed specifically to test the abilities associated with the criteria of understanding, appreciation, and reasoning. They also had three comparison groups matched to the study groups for age, gender, race, and socioeconomic status.

The results indicated that the proportion of subjects who scored in the impaired range was not significantly different across instruments and standards; however, a substantial number of subjects who performed adequately on one measure were found to have impaired performance on another. This finding suggested that those who do poorly on one standard will not necessarily do poorly on another, and choosing to use a single standard may not be warranted. Nor did the data support the notion of a hierarchy of stringency among the standards.

Given that the study suggested that each standard may identify partially distinct populations, using a combination of standards would produce a greater proportion of patients considered impaired in their decision-making capacities. In fact, Grisso and Appelbaum (1995a) reported that about 25% of their schizophrenic patients showed impaired judgment on any one measure, whereas more than 50% of them would be considered impaired if required to meet all three standards. The study therefore does not provide an answer to the question of where to fix the threshold of competence or incompetence, and perhaps there will never be a precise answer to this question. Grisso and Appelbaum (1998) recommended the four criteria that they have articulated as a focus for assessments of competence to consent to or refuse treatment. Future research may help to refine this focus, but for the moment it is clearly the most thoughtful and evidence-based one available.

Clinical Factors in the Approach to Assessing Decision-Making Capacity

The purpose of this chapter is not to provide a full account of the best approach to conducting an assessment of decision-making capacity. In this regard, the reader is referred to sources such as Grisso and Appelbaum (1998), Karel (2000), and Moye (2000), but a few points must be emphasized.

One is that (as noted in chapter 1) it is important to remain aware of the fact that in different segments of our pluralistic society, there may be different degrees of interest in the individual as an autonomous decision maker. A second is that patients who are seriously ill and dying are typically on many kinds of medications, some of which (e.g., certain analgesics) may cloud the patient's mental state and affect judgment (Werth, Benjamin, & Farrenkopf, 2000). A third is that the criteria for decision-making capacity, as articulated earlier, clearly indicate that a heavy emphasis is placed on the patient's cognitive ability, and less attention is paid to the influence of affect or affective states (Bursztajn, Harding, Gutheil, & Brodsky, 1991) or to the influence of health care values and beliefs (Karel, 2000). Unresolved grief, depression, or hypomanic denial can impair or distort cognitive processes and make it difficult to see the individual's baseline level of functioning. Both Bursztajn et al. (1991) and Appelbaum and Roth (1981) indicated that competency has too often been viewed as a fixed state, but, in fact, it may fluctuate with changes in the more basic mental and emotional attributes that underlie it. They recommended approaching the assessment of decision making as a dynamic process rather than as the application of a mere "test." This means understanding, for example, that intrapersonal and interpersonal issues as well as affective states can lead an individual to undervalue the positive outcomes of treatment. If these issues could be investigated and resolved, the patient might view his or her prospects in a different light.

On the issue of affective and dynamic influences, Sullivan and Youngner (1994) pointed out, however, that it seems inappropriate to assume that the mere presence of depression or any other psychological factor or conflict distorts a patient's decision-making capability. Assessments must be made on a case-by-case basis, and, in fact, the courts have not held that the simple presence of a mental or emotional disorder is sufficient to assume incompetence. The psychologist, then, must assess the patient's cognitive abilities to make decisions as well as weigh the influence exerted by affective and dynamic factors on the decision-making process. This challenging task, as Bursztajn et al. (1991) stated, should be "linked to an overall process designed to enhance the patient's autonomy" (p. 387) while attempting to ensure that reversible issues that distort judgment have been addressed and treated.

Methods of Assessing Decision-Making Capacity

There have been two methods of assessing decision making capacity: (a) assessment by interview, and (b) assessment by standardized instruments or tests. These different methods each have their strengths and weaknesses and might best be thought of as complementary to each other.

Assessment by Interview

Traditionally, the clinical assessment of decision-making capacity was relatively unstructured, but started with careful history taking and a thorough mental status examination (MSE). It also relied heavily on the acumen of the clinician. The MSE was considered useful in evaluating some of the cognitive functions that underlie decision making as well as determining whether evidence of a psychiatric disorder was present that might seriously affect decision-making capabilities (Farnsworth, 1990; Kaplan & Price, 1989; Searight, 1992). Some advocated for the inclusion of psychometric instruments (e.g., the Wechsler Adult Intelligence Scale) to test such functions as reasoning, memory, and judgment in a more standardized way (Bentivegna & Garvey, 1990).

This more traditional approach was questioned by those who held that the capacity to make health care decisions requires different functional abilities than those tested by the MSE or by psychological testing (Mishkin, 1989; Venesy, 1994). They stressed the importance of direct questioning about the patient's understanding and appreciation of the nature of his or her disorder, the recommended treatment, the risks and benefits involved, the alternatives, and their consequences.

The traditional interview approach has also been criticized as unreliable and lacking a clear consensus or gold standard (Moye, 2000). Grisso and Appelbaum (1998), in discussing the assessment of decision-making capacity by interview, also recommended that a structure such as that just noted be added to the interview. They have suggested that the evaluator approach the patient with the four criteria for competency (presented earlier) in mind and systematically question him or her relative to each of them. They further recommended retaining the MSE as part of the evaluation because of its value in detecting evidence of any possible mental disorder.

Assessment by Standardized Instruments

In recent years, standardized measures of decision-making capacity have been under development. The Hopkins Competency Assessment Test (HCAT; Janofsky, McCarthy, & Folstein, 1992) has been conceived as a tool for rapidly screening large numbers of patients for their competency to make treatment decisions and to write advance directives. The Competency Interview Schedule (CIS; Bean, Nishisato, Rector, & Glancey, 1994) has been devised to assess the decision-making ability of patients exploring the treatment option of electroconvulsive therapy. These two instruments are brief and easy to administer, but suffer from psychometric limitations. The HCAT tends to focus almost exclusively on only a single standard for determining competency: the ability to understand the relevant information involved in informed consent. The CIS is somewhat more comprehensive in that it incorporates items related to several standards, but it and the HCAT were both validated by comparing subjects' results with the global opinion of a clinician about competence or incompetence. The authors (Bean et al., 1994; Janofsky et al., 1992) provided little information about the standards of legal competency employed by the clinicians in their studies.

The use of clinical vignettes has been viewed as innovative and promising in terms of the development of competency assessment instruments. As Marson, Schmitt, Ingram, and Harrell (1994) noted, the clinical vignette is hypothetical, but can be made to closely approximate real-life situations. Marson, Ingram, Cody, and Harrell (1995) developed two specialized vignettes, one involving the case of a neoplasm and the other a case with a cardiac condition, that were designed to test the competency of patients with Alzheimer's disease under five legal standards. Vignettes such as these, with an operationalized scoring system, could prove to be very useful in assessing a patient's capacity to consent to treatment.

A far more complex and sophisticated effort at developing standardized and objectively scored measures of competence and incompetence was undertaken in the MacArthur Treatment Competence Study (Appelbaum & Grisso, 1995; Grisso, Appelbaum, Mulvey, & Fletcher, 1995; Grisso & Appelbaum, 1995b). The investigators in this study worked on developing reliable and valid measures of decision-making abilities that were conceptually related to the major legal standards for competence to consent to treatment. Three research instruments were constructed: (a) the Understanding Treatment Disclosures (UTD) instrument, (b) the Perceptions of Disorder (POD) instrument, and (c) the Thinking Rationally About Treatment (TRAT) instrument. Data on these three instruments were collected in a large, multisite study using samples of hospitalized patients with schizophrenia, major depression, and ischemic heart disease, as well as matched non-ill community samples. In a psychometrically sound manner, the authors examined scoring reliability, internal consistency, intertest correlations, test-retest correlations, and construct validity. They discussed and documented the psychometric strengths, weaknesses, and limitations of each instrument (Grisso et al., 1995; Grisso & Appelbaum, 1995b).

Because research demands required that these instruments be more lengthy and complex than desirable for clinical purposes, the principal authors have developed and validated an instrument designed for standardized clinical assessments of competence to consent to treatment (Grisso & Appelbaum, 1998). The MacArthur Competence Assessment Tool for Treatment Decisions (MacCAT-T) is based on the three instruments developed for the MacArthur Treatment Competence Study. The MacCAT-T is described as assessing abilities related to each of the four legal standards for competence, as requiring brief administration time, and as allowing the assessment of abilities in the context of the patient's own specific symptoms and treatment options.

Grisso and Appelbaum (1995b) cautioned that the measures that they developed should not be interpreted as though the measures, in themselves, can provide determinations of legal competence. As the investigators have said, no numerical criterion can give this sort of judgment across cases. Too many individual factors specific to each case need to be weighed in making a determination. As a result, they have suggested that those who score low on these standardized measures be considered as *at greater risk* of not meeting the legal criteria for competency. As Moye (2000) pointed out, the outcome of an assessment of this sort is not the test score per se, but the interpretation of the test score in the context of the many factors (e.g., educational, cultural, and ethnic differences) that may influence performance on standardized tests.

The Issue of Decision-Making Capacity in Special Populations

As Kleespies and Mori (1998) noted, several special populations of patients can present particular challenges in terms of determining their decision-making capacity. These include patients who are mentally ill, have dementia, are children or adolescents, or are developmentally disabled.

Mentally Ill Patients

As noted earlier, it was unfortunately common practice in the past to consider mentally ill patients as incompetent, particularly those with major mental illnesses. In more recent years, however, forensic experts and the courts have maintained that little substantial support exists for the position that psychiatric patients necessarily need protection from making incompetent decisions that differ from the protection given to medical patients when they consent to or refuse treatment (Cournos, 1993).

Yet in the MacArthur Treatment Competence Study noted earlier, Grisso and Appelbaum (1995b) found that the schizophrenia group had much higher proportions in the impaired categories on all three measures of decision-making capacity (UTD, POD, and TRAT) than either the depressive group or the ischemic heart disease group. Approximately, one quarter of the schizophrenia sample was found to be impaired on each measure, and when all three measures were used, 52% of the schizophrenia sample scored in the impaired range. Likewise, when combining all three measures, a greater proportion of the depressive sample scored in the impaired range than did the angina sample. Based on this sample, patients with mental illness could be said to manifest decision-making deficits more often than medically ill patients and their non-ill controls.

Grisso and Applebaum (1995b) pointed out, however, that considerable variability was found within and across the schizophrenia and depression groups. In fact, on any given measure, the majority of patients with schizophrenia did not do worse than other patients and nonpatients. The poorer mean performance of the schizophrenia group was attributable to a minority within that group, and the minority tended to be those who manifested more severe psychopathology (especially those with an acute thought disorder). The investigators concluded that significant differences seem to exist in decision-making abilities between persons with and without mental illness, but one cannot maintain from their data that all persons with mental illness lack decision-making abilities. In effect, it seems that each case must be evaluated on an individual basis.

Dementia Patients

Much the same can be said for patients with dementia. Both Stanley (1983) and Marson et al. (1994) stated that a diagnosis of dementia should not be taken as presumptive evidence of impaired decisional capacity. Dementia can be caused by various diseases, Alzheimer's disease being the most common. With Alzheimer's dementia, the onset of the illness is typically slow and a gradual decline in memory and cognitive functioning takes place. In the earliest stages of the disease, deficits may be mild and considerable cognitive ability may be retained. With multi-infarct dementia, the onset is typically more abrupt and more of a step-wise decline may occur. Initially, however, many of the person's cognitive functions may be relatively unimpaired and a recovery of functions can occur, something that is not seen in Alzheimer's dementia (Stanley, 1983).

Because such variations in the cognitive capacities of dementia patients can be identified, Marson et al. (1994) argued that a determination of decisional capacity should always involve a functional analysis of the patient. Neuropsychological and mental status test measures are clearly important in gauging the level of cognitive impairment, but, again, the findings from such testing must be linked to the kinds of capacities with which the law is concerned, that is, understanding, appreciation, and rational thinking.

An important concern with dementia patients has to do with the patient's ability to retain information over time. Stanley (1983) argued that it is not necessary to retain all consent information, but if retention is a serious concern, the patient should be re-evaluated on repeated occasions.

Given that Alzheimer's dementia can have a rather insidious progression, cases frequently occur in which the patient's decisional capacity seems to be in the borderline range. In the interest of promoting autonomous decision making for as long as possible in such cases, Stanley (1983) advocated that the process of informed consent be altered to accommodate the patient's needs. Thus, she has suggested such steps as making the consent material more readable, allowing the patient more time to review the consent material, using teaching and review methods, involving family members who may be able to use language that is more familiar to the patient, and so forth. In these ways, the dementia patient's ability to exercise autonomous decision making can be respected and optimized until the disease becomes too debilitating.

Children and Adolescents

The general rule of law with regard to children or minors is that they are legally incompetent to make medical decisions on their own behalf (Sigman & O'Connor, 1991). Parental consent is required for either treatment or the refusal of treatment, and parents are to be guided by the ethical principle of promoting their child's best interests. The American Academy of Pediatrics, however, has emphasized that "physicians and parents should give great weight to clearly expressed views of child patients regarding LSMT (life sustaining medical treatment), regardless of the legal particulars" (Committee on Bioethics, 1994, p. 532). Moreover, with adolescents, the parental consent requirement can have two exceptions.

The first exception is for *emancipated minors*. Emancipation means that the parents have relinquished control and authority over an adolescent who usually is living apart and is financially independent. Other circumstances that may be interpreted as indicating emancipation are marriage, military service, pregnancy, or parenthood. According to Sigman and O'Connor (1991), the emancipated minor exception has long been recognized as a common law rule and statutes in approximately half the states define circumstances under which a minor may be partially or wholly emancipated from his or her parents.

The second possible exception to the parental consent requirement has to do with the so-called *mature minor* doctrine. According to many courts, some state legislatures, and common law, adolescents who are 14 years of age or older can be assessed as sufficiently mature to make medical decisions for themselves (Committee on Bioethics, 1994; Sigman & O'Connor, 1991). Mature in this case means being able to understand the nature of an illness and the nature and consequences of accepting or refusing the proposed medical treatment. Traditionally, the courts have viewed the age of 14 as the cutoff for the application of this doctrine, and some empirical evidence supports this point of view. Weithorn and Campbell (1982), for example, presented 9, 14, 18, and 21-year-olds with hypothetical treatment dilemmas and found that while 9-year-olds appeared to be less competent according to legal standards, 14-year-olds did not differ from the 18 and 21-year-olds. Studies such as this one, however, need to be carefully validated before conclusions are drawn.

The mature minor doctrine remains shrouded in legal uncertainty. According to Sigman and O'Connor (1991), the courts have allowed physicians to act with impunity on the decisions of minors when the intervention entailed small risk (e.g., a tonsillectomy). When a major medical intervention or a refusal of life-sustaining treatment was at issue, however, either a court order has been required or the assent of a parent to the minor's decision.

Developmentally Disabled Patients

Some have argued that mild mental retardation does not preclude good judgment and decision making with regard to specific decisions about treatment (Kaplan, Strang, & Ahmed, 1988). Clearly, all efforts should be made to respect the autonomy of such patients in the informed consent process. Patients who are considered more seriously developmentally disabled or suffer from moderate to severe mental retardation, however, may never have had any hope of attaining decision-making capacity or competency. Some of these individuals live with parents or their legal guardians, while others are wards of the state and live in public facilities. The state has a special interest in and responsibility for the protection of these vulnerable people.

In the past, a few courts argued for the extension of the right to refuse life-sustaining treatment even to those patients, such as developmentally disabled patients, who have never attained the competency to express treatment preferences. They typically proposed that the patient might exercise this right through a surrogate who used substituted judgment. With the realization, however, that it would be impossible for a surrogate to formulate a substituted judgment for someone who has never been competent to express treatment preferences, the best interests standard has replaced substituted judgment in court proceedings.

McKnight and Bellis (1992) asserted that developmentally disabled patients do not have the right to refuse life-sustaining treatment, but they clearly have a right to have appropriate medical decisions made on their behalf. They have proposed that a legally appointed primary decision maker might choose to forego life-sustaining treatment for a developmentally disabled person in situations such as a persistent vegetative state, a terminal illness with uncontrollable pain, and so forth. In each situation, they hold that the best interests standard is to be applied and that the focus should be on the value of continuing life for the individual patient. They have cautioned, and rightly so, that this population must be protected from societal and financial pressures, and McKnight and Bellis have proposed that any consideration of the cost of life-sustaining treatment be prohibited in the process of making these decisions.

CONCLUSION

This chapter reviews the ethical and legal foundations for end-of-life decision making. Under American law, autonomy or self-determination and its derivative, the doctrine of informed consent, seem to have carried the day. It should be evident, however, that our society's recent, more definitive embrace of the ethical and legal principle of autonomy in end-of-life decision making does not mean that all is settled or well understood when it comes to its application in particular cases. Nor can it be said that the concept of patient self-determination has fully penetrated the health care system. Many instances of medical paternalism still appear in which patients' wishes are not attended to or are frankly disregarded (Asch, Hansen-Flaschen, & Lanken, 1995). Thus, the ethical and legal status of end-of-life care must be regarded as still evolving and developing, or as work in progress. Chapter 3 proceeds to examine those potential choices or options that have been ethically and legally sanctioned by our society for those with a terminal illness.

3

THE WISH TO DIE: DECISIONS THAT DO NOT PROLONG OR MAY HASTEN THE DYING PROCESS

Death is not the worst; rather, in vain
To wish for death, and not to compass it.

—Sophocles, *Electra*, l, 1008

For many elderly terminally ill patients, particularly for those nearing the
end of a chronic, progressive, ultimately fatal disease, the time and manner of death can, to a certain extent, result from a choice.

—Finucane and Harper, 1996, p. 369

As the Institute of Medicine's Committee on Care at the End of Life
has stated, physicians and hospitals in the United States regulate many
aspects of life's beginning and ending, "sometimes excessively so" (Field &
Cassel, 1997, p. 50). The Committee's statement has been a clear acknowledgment that technological approaches to medical conditions have their limits and can have a negative impact when more personal and empathic care is
needed. With regard to the birth process, the Committee noted that the
increased use of childbirth classes, an increased interest in assistance from
midwives, a more selective use of medications, and the development of
birthing centers have reflected a reaction to medicine's increasingly technological orientation to the management of labor and delivery. With respect to

the process of dying, the emergence of the hospice movement with its emphasis on comfort care at the end of life, the formation of organizations such as Compassion in Dying and the Hemlock Society that have been associated with the so-called *right to die* movement, the enactment of the Patient Self-Determination Act of 1990, and the passage of the Oregon Death with Dignity Act (ODDA) clearly indicate that efforts have been made to counteract the use of high-tech approaches to prolonging, unnecessarily, the lives of terminally ill patients who wish to die.

The same forces (noted in chapter 1) that have driven concern about quality of life, as well as the quest for death with dignity, have also driven the hospice movement and the right to die movement. These forces include the increased frequency of a prolonged but debilitating illness at the end of life, the ability of high-tech medicine to sustain life, although it may have become relatively meaningless, and the often impersonal nature of dying in institutions such as hospitals and nursing homes. Proponents of these disparate movements have advocated for increased self-determination in the dying process and decreased control of dying by physicians and medical institutions. In this chapter, our discussion will focus on those now accepted health care practices in which the patient may exercise some choice either not to prolong life or, in some respects, to follow a course that indirectly may hasten death. These practices have to do with the refusal of life-sustaining treatment, the use of medications or procedures to relieve pain and suffering that may also have the effect of bringing about an earlier death, and the extension, through advance care planning, of the patient's right to make such choices even when he or she is no longer competent to make a decision. The chapter that follows this one (chapter 4) will deal with those practices such as assisted suicide and euthanasia that are more controversial and not widely accepted practices in the United States.

THE REFUSAL OF LIFE-SUSTAINING TREATMENT

Withdrawing and Withholding Treatment

Withdrawing and withholding life-sustaining treatment is a legally protected means for those who are considered terminally ill and want to exercise some choice over the time and circumstances of their death. Included among those technologically assisted treatments that are considered life sustaining are (a) the use of respirators and endotracheal intubation for breathing difficulties, (b) intravenous feeding for nutrition and hydration problems, (c) hemodialysis for kidney failure, (d) radiation and chemotherapy to impede the growth of cancer, (e) cardiopulmonary resuscitation (CPR), and (f) the implantation of a defibrillator or a pacemaker for cardiac problems. In effect, life-sustaining treatment can be taken to mean any medical intervention that would have little or no effect on the underlying disease, injury, or condition, but is administered to forestall the time of death or to reinstate life when death can be regarded as having occurred (Hafemeister, Keilitz, & Banks, 1991; Maddi, 1990; McKnight & Bellis, 1992).

The legal basis of the right to refuse life-sustaining treatment has been discussed in chapter 2. Acceptance of this right is now widespread in the United States, and so, for example, it is currently not uncommon to have Do Not Resuscitate (DNR) or Do Not Intubate (DNI) orders for terminally ill patients in hospitals and nursing homes. It is important to remember, however, that historically this acceptance has been achieved over a relatively short period of time. In 1976, the medical staff caring for Karen Ann Quinlan (who was in an irreversible state of unconsciousness) did not feel inclined or empowered to remove her from a ventilator, although her family had repeatedly requested that this be done (In re Quinlan, 1976). After the Quinlan family had obtained court approval and had the ventilator disconnected, Ms. Quinlan lived on, still in an unconscious state, for another 8 years while she received artificial nutrition and hydration. She finally died of pneumonia. As recently as the mid-1980s, it required a California Court of Appeals decision before a competent, terminally ill patient could be removed from a mechanical ventilator at his own request (Bartling v. Superior Court, 1984).

Although medical ethicists have long equated withholding and withdrawing life-sustaining treatment, some evidence has suggested that physicians may have a preference for withholding treatment as opposed to starting and then withdrawing it (Committee on Bioethics, 1994; Singer, 1992; Snyder & Swartz, 1993). In this regard, one view is that it may be easier psychologically if the physician maintains a more passive role in allowing the patient to die rather than stopping a treatment that will result in the patient's death (McCamish & Crocker, 1993). Burns, Mitchell, Griffith, and Truog (2001) found that, in a sample of pediatric critical care practitioners, those with less experience were more likely to be reluctant to withdraw life-sustaining treatment. They suggested that those with less experience were possibly less familiar and less comfortable with the issues involved. A potential risk of preferentially withholding rather than withdrawing treatment, however, is that some patients may be subtly influenced not to try a treatment they might find acceptable. A physician's willingness to withdraw treatment can allow for a time-limited trial in situations when the prognosis is uncertain or disagreement exists over a decision.

One of the most emotionally charged and debated issues related to refusing life-sustaining treatment has been withholding or withdrawing artificial nutrition and hydration (Boisaubin, 1993). Having adequate food and water is a very basic need, and providing food and drink to others is closely linked to caring and nurturance. It should come as no surprise then that withholding or withdrawing nutrition and hydration can be a very disturbing decision to make. The argument revolves around whether nutrition and hydration are regarded as basic needs or, when artificially given, are considered a medical treatment indistinguishable in any morally relevant way from other life-sustaining treatments (McCamish & Crocker, 1993).

In the *Cruzan* case mentioned in the preceding chapter, this issue, although not the main judicial focus, was nonetheless considered by the U.S. Supreme Court. The Court adopted the consensus opinion that artificial nutrition and hydration are life-sustaining, medical interventions to be treated no differently than other such interventions. This judicial opinion did not totally resolve the issue, however, because a few states continued to have laws that did not permit the refusal of nutrition and hydration (Snyder & Swartz, 1993). Moreover, with respect to children, Congress passed Public Law 98–457 (1984), the *Child Abuse Prevention and Treatment and Adoption Reform Act* (commonly referred to as the *Baby Doe Rules*), which requires that artificial feeding be continued for children even in terminal conditions (Boisaubin, 1993). Given these apparent differences between the judicial and legislative branches of government, the issue of withdrawing or withholding artificial nutrition with children who are dying does not appear to be settled.

Unresolved Issues in the Refusal of Life-Sustaining Treatment

Given the recentness and complexity of these changes in practice, it is not surprising that issues related to refusing life-sustaining treatment remain unresolved. Thus, no real consensus has yet been made on such critical issues as a medical definition of "terminal" if a time frame is included in the definition (Powell & Cohen, 1994) or, as we have seen in chapter 2, on the criteria for mental competence to make decisions. Also, no consensus has been reached on how someone can best represent the interests of those most vulnerable patients, the incompetent terminally ill who have no family or friends to act as surrogates.

With regard to terminal illness, a definition found with some frequency is that an illness is considered *terminal* when it has a predictably fatal outcome and no known cure exists. Often this definition has been set within a time frame and is limited to cases in which death was thought to be expected within 6 months. Increasingly, however, it has been acknowledged that medicine is not an exact science, and it is often difficult to predict with accuracy when a patient will die (Maddi, 1990; Mishara, 1999; Thibault, 1997). Christakis and Lamont (2000), for example, found that 63% of doctors, when asked for prognoses upon referring patients to a hospice program, were overoptimistic in their predictions for survival. Only 20% of the physicians were accurate (with accuracy defined as between .67 and 1.33 times the actual length of survival), and 17% were overpessimistic.

Findings such as these have led the Committee on Care at the End of Life (Field & Cassel, 1997) to refer to the prediction of the course of an illness and remaining life expectancy as "an exercise in uncertainty" (p. 30). In effect, it may be less misleading if the definition of terminal illness is not quite so locked into a time frame, or if, as Lynn (2001) suggested, it is taken as applicable when the individual is sufficiently ill that dying this year would not be a surprise. Yet many patients and treatment providers remain bound by the fact that obtaining Medicare coverage for hospice services still requires a determination that the patient has a life expectancy of 6 months or less.

A number of efforts have been made to develop models to predict the likelihood of survival for critically ill patients. The Acute Physiology, Age, and Chronic Health Evaluation (APACHE) methodology is perhaps the best known of these systems, and APACHE III represents its third revision (Knaus et al., 1991). Thibault (1997), however, pointed out some of the limitations of such statistical models. As he has noted, they produce probability estimates that were developed and validated on large patient populations. Thus, the model might predict 50% mortality for the next 100 intensive care unit (ICU) patients and be absolutely correct that 50% will die. Yet it cannot predict which 50 individuals will die. In attempting to predict individual patient mortality, the model could potentially be absolutely incorrect and predict the wrong 50 patients. On the individual predictive level, typically only a relatively few patients are at the extreme of a very high risk of death. It is therefore difficult to achieve the sample size that would provide the statistical stability needed to make predictions with a high degree of accuracy. Thibault concludes that "we are far from achieving the goal of using individual patient predictors to make the difficult and painful decisions regarding which critically ill patients may no longer benefit from intensive care" (p. 361).

The question of the criteria for determining the capacity to refuse treatment has been discussed in detail in chapter 2. In brief, Grisso and Appelbaum (1998) proposed four criteria for determining decision-making capabilities, and they have developed an assessment instrument that is very helpful in evaluating patients on each criterion. The four criteria are (a) the ability to express a choice, (b) the ability to understand information relevant to the decision about treatment, (c) the ability to appreciate the significance of the information disclosed for one's own illness and possible treatment, and (d) the ability to reason with relevant information in order to engage in a logical process of weighing treatment options. Legal authorities and those responsible for treating terminally ill patients may eventually adopt these four criteria as the standards for making a determination of competency. At present, however, no clearly stated consensus has been established on this issue, and different states and jurisdictions may use one of these criteria or some combination of two or three. As mentioned in chapter 2, whether one uses one, two, or four criteria can make a difference in the threshold for competence and incompetence. A higher threshold may mean that more patients are denied the opportunity for autonomous decision making, while a lower threshold may mean that some vulnerable patients are not protected from their impaired decision-making abilities. Obviously, it behooves the clinician to know which criteria or standards are typically employed in the jurisdiction in which he or she practices.

The cases of *Quinlan* and *Cruzan* have illustrated (even though it was not the main point of contention in each case) the struggle over the question of who is appropriate to make decisions about withholding or withdrawing treatment when the patient is no longer capable of doing so. In these particular cases, family members were recognized in the judicial process as appropriate surrogate decision makers for the incompetent patient if no health care proxy or guardian had previously been appointed. A greater problem arises, however, with those patients who are terminally ill, incompetent, and have no family or friends to act as surrogates. It would not seem to be in keeping with the value that our society has placed on autonomy to take the position that these individuals have somehow forfeited their right to have a surrogate decision maker to attempt to exercise substituted judgment or at least someone to advocate for their best interests. Efforts to resolve this difficult dilemma are discussed in a later section of this chapter (see "End-of-Life Decisions in the Absence of Advance Directives").

Does the Refusal of Life-Sustaining Treatment Constitute Suicide?

Given issues such as those mentioned earlier, some have had reservations about how the right to refuse life-sustaining treatment is implemented. Still others, because of their particular mores or values, have wondered if it constitutes *suicide* on the part of the patient. Mayo's position (Mayo, 1992) might be interpreted as compatible with such ideas, but Mayo also would not assume that all suicides are immoral, blameworthy, or in need of intervention, particularly not those of terminally ill patients who are suffering without relief, who have very poor quality of life, and who wish to die. His perspective is that "much of the controversy in the literature about euthanasia and suicide (and about the definitions thereof) is obfuscated by the suspicious premise that anything that can be labeled 'suicide' is to be condemned, discouraged, pitied, or treated" (Mayo, 1992, p. 91).

Mayo (1992) defined suicide as ending one's life intentionally. Given that refusing life-sustaining treatment might be viewed as bringing about one's end intentionally, it could be considered consistent with his definition. The issue of whether the refusal of life-sustaining treatment constitutes suicide, however, becomes complicated when one takes into account certain situational variables.

For example, recipients of life-sustaining treatments may include patients who are having multisystem failures and are kept alive on a ventilator with seemingly very poor quality of life, as well as patients with end-stage renal disease (ESRD) who are maintained with dialysis treatments and seemingly have the opportunity for a relatively good quality of life. As noted earlier, life-sustaining treatment can be taken to mean any medical intervention that would have little or no effect on the underlying disease, injury, or condition, but is administered to forestall the time of death. In the case of the patient on the ventilator, it would seem that meaningful life is essentially coming to an end and the refusal of further treatment is closer to what Parry (1990) and McCamish and Crocker (1993) referred to as allowing the underlying disease or condition to take over. Farrenkopf and Bryan (1999) characterized such a case as an attempt to exercise some control of the dying process. Allowing oneself to die when life is basically over would hardly seem to have the same connotations as is typically ascribed to the term *suicide*, particularly because suicide so frequently involves cutting short a still viable life. On the other hand, if the dialysis patient, who seemed to have the opportunity for meaningful life, were to find the intrusive and restricting interventions of dialysis unacceptable and choose to forego them, it would seem to be more conceivably within the parameters of what has been referred to as "preemptive suicide" (Cohen, Steinberg, Hails, Dobscha, & Fischel, 2000, p. 196).

These are complicated issues, and certain situations seem to defy easy definition. The same may be said, however, for the issue of whether withdrawing life-sustaining treatment is a form of so-called *passive* euthanasia.

Does the Withholding or Withdrawal of Life-Sustaining Treatment Constitute Passive Euthanasia?

The withholding and withdrawal of life-sustaining treatment has been referred to by some as *passive euthanasia* (e.g., Colt, 1991). The term *euthanasia*, of course, has had a number of meanings over the centuries. Its origins are Greek, and in ancient times it meant literally a *good death*. It subsequently has been used to refer to the taking of a life to end unbearable suffering. In the 20th century, however, euthanasia was also used in reference to the sinister practice of mass murder employed in the World War II era Nazi death camps. For some, such a connotation still seems to be associated with the term, and that being the case, it is unfortunate that it occasionally has been applied to withholding or withdrawing life-sustaining treatment for terminally ill patients.

Clinicians and ethicists have clearly distinguished between *killing* and *allowing to die* (McCamish & Crocker, 1993). The withholding and withdrawal of life-sustaining treatment, when done with the informed consent of the terminally ill patient or his or her surrogate, falls within the realm of allowing to die. Allowing to die in this context essentially means that life-sustaining treatment is withheld or withdrawn with the agreement of the patient or surrogate, and the underlying disease or condition is permitted to cause death. The patient dies as he or she would have without the use of support technology.

A problem arises when the decision to withhold or withdraw life-sustaining treatment is made without the knowledge or consent of the patient or his or her surrogate. Somewhat alarmingly, the survey by Asch, Hansen-Flaschen, and Lanken (1995) left little doubt that this sometimes happens. In order to determine practices with regard to limiting life-sustaining treatment, these investigators surveyed a national sample of 879 physicians who practiced in adult ICUs in the United States. They found that 23% of this sample of critical care physicians had withheld or withdrawn life-sustaining treatment without the consent of the patient or his or her surrogate. Moreover, 12% had withheld or withdrawn treatment without the knowledge of the patient or the surrogate. These decisions were based on the physician's judgment that further treatment was futile.

It would be very problematic if decisions such as those noted were made unilaterally and had to do with treatments that others might judge to be potentially beneficial. Asch et al. have concluded that the survey findings "may be a disturbing sign of paternalism" (p. 291). Not only are they ethically questionable, but given that these determinations were made extrajudicially, their legal status would seem to be uncertain (Nicholson & Matross, 1989). The findings seem to call for further inquiry as well as an increased emphasis on oversight in combination with the use of guidelines to assist clinicians who are in the position of making such decisions. Because most hospitals currently have policy and procedure statements that provide for oversight and guidelines on this topic, it would seem to be a matter of insisting that these policies and procedures are observed by those making the immediate patient care decisions.

INTERVENTIONS THAT MAY HASTEN DEATH

The term *interventions that may hasten death* is used advisedly here. In some sense, all decisions that either foreshorten the time of death, or prevent or interrupt a process that might prolong life, might be viewed as decisions or interventions that *hasten death*. These would include decisions to withhold or withdraw life-sustaining treatment, pain relief under the principle of the double effect, terminal sedation, terminal dehydration, assisted suicide, and so forth. As the APA Working Group (2000) pointed out, however, many would disagree with such an inclusive frame of reference. Such disagreements have stemmed from differences about whether interventions like withdrawing life-sustaining treatment can be seen as, in any way, similar to an intervention like assisted suicide.

The preceding section of this chapter discusses withholding and withdrawing life-sustaining treatment. In the current section, the focus of discussion is on those other interventions or decisions that indirectly may hasten death and are generally considered acceptable practice in the United States. As noted earlier, a discussion of the more controversial topics of assisted suicide and euthanasia will be reserved for chapter 4.

The Relief of Pain and the Principle of the Double Effect

The principle of the double effect is often raised in bioethical discussions of interventions that may indirectly hasten death (Battin, 1994; Kleespies, Hughes, & Gallacher, 2000; Mayo, 1992). As mentioned in chapter 2, this ethical principle is taken as justification for performing an act that has a foreseen negative effect (e.g., death) as long as one does not intend the negative effect and only intends a positive effect (e.g., relief from otherwise intractable pain). As cited in Battin (1994, p. 17), the following four conditions are necessary to meet the criteria for this principle:

(1) the action must not be intrinsically wrong; (2) the agent must intend only the good effect, not the bad one; (3) the bad effect must not be the means of achieving the good effect; and (4) the good effect must be "proportional" to the bad one, that is, outweigh it.

When applied to decisions about the care of a terminally ill patient, it permits a physician, for example, to prescribe increasing doses of analgesics and sedatives with the intention of easing pain and suffering, although a secondary effect might be the slowing of respirations and ending life more quickly. In such a case, the intent is to relieve suffering, not to kill the patient or to assist the patient in committing suicide.

Invoking the principle of the double effect has been challenged from two directions. First, Fohr (1998) maintained that little evidence suggests that the appropriate titration of opioid analgesics hastens death. In fact, she has argued that reference to the double effect argument in relation to pain medication, such as morphine, only heightens the fears of the medical staff that they are killing the patient and consequently leads to the undertreatment of pain.

Second, whether a physician can always maintain a clear distinction between intentions has been questioned by Quill (1993) and Quill, Dresser, and Brock (1997). These authors argued that the principle of the double effect is an idealized and superficial view of human intent, which is often quite complex and, at times, even contradictory. They believe that the rule of the double effect is rigid, procrustean, and fails to acknowledge the real-life ambiguities of intentionality. Battin (1994), for example, claimed that it is implausible to imagine that intelligent individuals would not be conscious of both the primary and secondary effects of their decisions, especially if one of those effects is as significant as death. Therefore, it could hardly be said that they would not intend for such an effect to occur. According to this perspective, the physician who prescribes increasing doses of analgesics and sedatives may well intend, at some level, both pain management and a hastening of death.

In fact, some evidence for this position can be found in a small study on the use of sedatives and analgesics during the withholding and withdrawal of life-sustaining treatment (Wilson, Smedira, Fink, McDowell, & Luce, 1992). In this investigation, the researchers found that physicians ordered and nurses administered such medications with the intention of hastening death in nearly 40% of the critically ill patients in their sample, but in no instance was it the only reason given for doing so. The physicians and nurses concurrently cited relief of pain, anxiety, or air hunger as reasons for using this type of medication.

Those who hold this latter position do not see such hastened or assisted deaths as necessarily immoral or unethical because instances of both can be shown to promote human dignity rather than destroy it. In this regard, they often cite the coup de grace granted a mortally wounded soldier who cannot be saved on the battlefield or an abortion to save the life of a mother (Battin, 1994).

Proponents of the double effect argument, however, have steadfastly maintained that it is possible to draw a clear distinction between "intended results and unintended but accepted consequences" (Annas, 1996, p. 685). As noted in chapter 2, the U.S. Supreme Court in the cases of *Washington v. Glucksberg* (1997) and *Vacco v. Quill* (1997) appears to have agreed with this position. Moreover, in a study of end-of-life care in a pediatric ICU after the withdrawal of life-sustaining treatment, Burns et al. (2000) found that the staff was in near-universal agreement on the use of sedatives or analgesics to decrease pain, anxiety, and air hunger, even though they might hasten death. The staff in this investigation perceived hastening death as an acceptable but unintended side effect; that is, they employed the double effect principle to justify their actions. The authors concluded that, in the absence of a viable alternative, double effect reasoning provided a rationale for clinicians who neither supported euthanasia on the one hand nor the practice of allowing patients to die with untreated suffering on the other. Yet given the evidence presented by Fohr (1998) and the findings of Wilson et al. (1992) noted earlier, the dispute over whether this rationale is necessary or sufficient hardly seems settled.

Terminal Sedation

Terminal sedation refers to the use of high doses of sedatives to render a consenting patient unconscious as a means of relieving extremes of intractable physical pain and suffering, such as in cases of severe headache secondary to swelling of the brain (Quill & Byock, 2000). Again, as mentioned in chapter 2, the Supreme Court decisions noted earlier (i.e., *Glucksberg* and *Vacco*) have also been interpreted as extending approval to this practice as a last resort for those who are dying and suffering unbearably without relief. Justices O'Connor and Souter wrote concurrences to these decisions that have suggested that the practice is permissible under current law.

In the context of imminent death, terminal sedation can be achieved with a barbiturate or benzodiazepine infusion that is rapidly increased until a level of sedation eliminates signs of pain and discomfort. This state is then maintained until the patient dies. Truog, Berde, Mitchell, and Grier (1992) commented that the use of barbiturates for this purpose may be ethically troubling to some because barbiturates are not analgesics and have been used for lethal purposes. For patients in severe pain, they recommend maintaining opioid infusions along with barbiturates to minimize any possible pain. Although barbiturates and other sedating medications may hasten death, Truog et al. and Quill and Byock (2000) viewed their use as ethically justifiable in dosages that sedate but are not lethal per se. The main indications for terminal sedation have been to relieve severe physical suffering when all reasonable alternatives have failed, and to produce unconsciousness before terminal extubation from a ventilator so the patient does not experience agonal respirations or air hunger.

When a patient is suffering greatly, when he or she has no real prospects of recovery, and when terminal sedation is considered, the circumstances are typically such that the patient or patient's surrogate has consented to withhold and withdraw life-prolonging measures, such as artificial nutrition or hydration and antibiotics. Given that, under these cumulative circumstances, death is a foreseeable, perhaps inevitable, outcome of the patient's condition plus the sedating medication, Quill and Byock (2000) noted that "the act can be more morally complex and ambiguous than is often acknowledged" (p. 409). Orentlicher (1997), in fact, referred to it as "essentially euthanasia" (p. 1239). In effect, as Truog et al. (1992) stated, the hastening of death in such extreme cases is often seen as a "blessing" for the patient.

Although they have acknowledged that cases like this strain the boundaries of the principle of the double effect, Krakauer et al. (2000) have argued that a difference exists between terminal sedation and euthanasia. The difference is said to hinge on whether or not the medications are being titrated to comfort the patient. Thus, it is argued that if the physician is titrating the medications to comfort, he or she does not intend the patient's death.

Terminal Dehydration

With terminal dehydration, a terminally ill patient who is competent and otherwise physically able to take nourishment makes a voluntary decision to refuse food and fluids, and is allowed to die a gradual death (Miller & Meier, 1998; Quill & Byock, 2000; Quill, Lo, & Brock, 1997). As a method of dying, it does not require any physician's involvement in directly or intentionally hastening death. It is said that such a death is not painful and that discomfort from the process itself, as well as from the underlying disease, can be managed with standard palliative measures, including terminal sedation as a last resort. The process is made somewhat easier by the fact that, in the course of events with many terminal illnesses, patients often lose their appetite and greatly decrease their food and fluid intake. Ethically and legally, the cessation of *natural* eating and drinking has been considered an extension of the now established right to refuse artificial nutrition and hydration under similar circumstances. On the other hand, such an action or, more precisely, inaction seems to challenge or actually blur the distinction between the refusal of life-sustaining treatment and suicide. As noted earlier, Mayo's definition of suicide (Mayo, 1992) is ending one's life intentionally. Suicide can be accomplished by intentional inaction as well as by doing something more active. In ceasing to eat and drink, the patient brings about his or her own death by dehydration.

Despite these potential moral complexities, this manner of death has been widely accepted by hospice and palliative care physicians (Quill, Lo, & Brock, 1997). As Miller and Meier (1998) indicated, terminal dehydration can be made painless but not swift. Depending on the patient's nutritional and metabolic state and the overall burden of his or her disease, dying can take anywhere from several days to 3 or 4 weeks. Dying in this manner requires considerable determination and resolve on the part of the patient to continue his or her fast. It is a method that is available to all competent, suffering patients, but it is clearly not something that everyone would want to try. A supportive family and clinical staff that provide good palliative care would seem to be crucial to such an effort, but as Quill, Lo, and Brock (1997) noted, the notion of allowing a patient to dehydrate or starve to death may nonetheless seem repugnant to many. Patients, for example, can go into a confused or delirious state, something that can erode their wish to have a dignified death. If the patient is confused, questions can arise as to whether his or her decision remains voluntary. In short, much is still unknown about this option. At present, little information is available, other than that obtained through anecdotal accounts, about how frequently terminal patients choose this manner of death; which patients make such a choice; how often they are successful in carrying it through to the end; what the emotional costs and benefits are for the patient, staff, and family; and so forth. Moreover, as mentioned earlier, the ethical and moral implications do not seem to have been fully explored.

THE STRUGGLE TO DECIDE

As is evident, the choices for the patient who is near the end of life, or his or her surrogate's choices, are often ethically complicated. They are also highly emotion laden. They involve letting go of life and loved ones. They also involve cultural, religious, and personal values and beliefs about life and death.

The psychologist and other health providers can review helpful information with the patient and his or her family when they are struggling with these difficult decisions. Such information has been clearly presented in everyday language in booklets such as *Hard Choices for Loving People* by Dunn (1994). In his booklet, Dunn explained that for frail, elderly, sick patients who have a cardiac arrest, CPR has a rather low success rate and can carry some very significant potential burdens. Thus, Tresch et al. (1993) studied 196 nursing home residents who sustained a cardiac arrest and received CPR from paramedics. Of this group, 19% were successfully resuscitated and hospitalized, but only 5% survived to be discharged from the hospital. Awoke, Mouton, and Parrott (1992) did a retrospective chart review of 45 elderly residents of a long-term care facility who received CPR from in-house physicians. Nine residents (20%) were successfully resuscitated, but 7 of these died within 24 hours of hospitalization and none survived to return to long-term care. In another study, Tresch et al. (1994) reviewed the cases of hospitalized patients who experienced a cardiac arrest and received CPR. Of this group, a higher percentage (26%) survived to be discharged, but the higher survival rate was attributed to a greater selectivity about which patients would benefit from resuscitation attempts (Schwenzer, Smith, & Durbin, 1993).

It is noteworthy that, for those who survive, the force applied during CPR may result in broken ribs or even a punctured lung. If the patient is without oxygen for any significant amount of time, brain damage can occur. Moreover, some patients may need to be placed on a ventilator for continued survival, even though such an event might not have been something they would have wanted. Such suffering can be averted if a carefully weighed decision is made to have a DNR order written by a physician so that CPR is withheld.

As mentioned earlier, it can be a difficult decision to withhold or withdraw artificially administered nutrition and hydration from a patient who is in the end stages of a terminal illness, yet feeding tubes themselves are not completely free from risks and burdens (Quill, 1989). If the tube is displaced or regurgitated fluid enters the lungs, pneumonia can develop. The constant rubbing of the tube can lead to ulcerations, and infections can occur. Patients often struggle to remove a feeding tube and need to be restrained. Such scenarios can be very unpleasant for the patient.

Patients who are in the end stages of a life-threatening illness typically have very little appetite and do not *starve* to death. Rather, they become dehydrated long before they suffer from lack of nourishment (Printz, 1992). It is important to know that the dry mouth and sense of thirst that accompany dehydration can be eased with good mouth care and with the use of ice chips or sips of water. To the greatest degree possible, any pain or discomfort can be medicated, but Printz (1992) also observed that dehydration appears to have an analgesic effect. Thus, withdrawing or withholding artificial nutrition and hydration, or any life-sustaining treatment, does not mean the end of care. It only means that the focus of care shifts to comfort care primarily.

The shift to comfort care for dying patients has been the approach advocated by the hospice movement and by palliative care programs. As Dunn (1994) noted, comfort measures include such things as medication for pain or fever reduction, or oxygen to make breathing easier. This approach also entails the elimination of cure-oriented treatments, procedures, and diagnostic tests, many of which involve some pain or discomfort in themselves. Thus, radiation or chemotherapy (with all their discomforting side effects) would be discontinued for the cancer patient unless, in the larger scheme of things, they provided some relief of the overall burden of pain. Likewise, surgery would not be performed unless it was necessary to relieve pain or to increase the patient's comfort. Thus, patients at times have the option to shift to comfort measures only and prevent a prolonged dying process. They also have the opportunity to assist their family, surrogate decision makers, and treatment providers by making their wishes about comfort care known, while they are still of sound mind, through a process of advance care planning. (See chapter 6 of this volume for a further discussion of the approach of hospice and palliative care.)

ADVANCE CARE PLANNING

In the preceding sections of this chapter, the ethically and legally accepted options available to the competent, terminally ill patient who does not wish to prolong life under intolerable conditions are discussed. As alluded to earlier, however, the need to make decisions about life-sustaining treatment or about events that may result in a hastened death often occurs after the disease has progressed to the point where the patient no longer has the capacity to participate meaningfully in the decision-making process. Self-determination, in such cases, is only realized for individuals who have expressed their wishes in advance, that is, while still competent. Advance care planning refers to the methods that might allow competent individuals to extend their autonomy into the future by permitting them to document their preferred approach to end-of-life care or to designate someone else to make their health care decisions in the event they are not able to do so for themselves. Although these methods are not always used to convey wishes to limit end-of-life care (e.g., they can be used to express a wish to have all possible end-of-life treatment), a discussion is included here because they are frequently used to curtail the unwanted prolongation of life.

By preserving the autonomy of the individual, the hope has been that advance care planning could help address the ethical and legal complications that often arise when incompetent individuals are faced with end-of-life treatment decisions. This issue has become increasingly salient to our society since the aforementioned *Quinlan* case, and it was most dramatically highlighted in the previously noted Supreme Court decision in the *Cruzan* case (refer to chapter 2). In the *Cruzan* case, it was established that an incompetent, terminally ill individual could forego life-sustaining treatment (with the decision of a surrogate), but that the state had the right to set evidentiary requirements for surrogate decision makers. In Missouri, this meant that the state could demand *clear and convincing evidence* that this is what the incompetent individual would have wanted if competent. Nancy Beth Cruzan's parents had to obtain the testimony of additional witnesses, who swore that she had stated to them prior to her injury that she would not want to live in a vegetative state. The state court then allowed her to be removed from life-sustaining treatment.

The Promotion of Advance Directives

Related to the *Cruzan* decision, the U.S. Supreme Court has strongly advocated the use of *advance directives* to protect the self-determination of individuals who have reached a point in their illness when they are no longer able to make their own decisions about their care (Wachter & Lo, 1993). An advance directive is a means of stating one's preferences for medical treatment while still mentally capable and in anticipation of a time when one will no longer be as capable.

Advance directives generally take two forms. One involves completing a document called a *living will* in which the individual specifies his or her treatment preferences for end-of-life care. It may specify certain conditions (e.g., a state of permanent unconsciousness) that the person might like managed in a particular way, or it might indicate whether or not the person would like particular treatments (e.g., artificial nutrition and hydration) to be withdrawn or maintained. A living will can be formal or informal; that is, it may be expressed in a legal document or in notes, letters, and oral statements to family, friends, and treatment providers.

A second form of advance directive involves identifying a person or surrogate to make decisions on one's behalf when one is no longer able to do so. Such a person is called a *health care proxy* or a *durable power of attorney for health care*. The proxy or surrogate decision maker is generally expected to be guided by a *substituted judgment* standard (i.e., to attempt to make the decision that the incompetent person would make if competent). If that is not possible, the person is to be guided by a *best interests* standard in which he or she considers the highest net benefit to the individual in question, given the available options and the person's known preferences and values (Beauchamp & Childress, 2001).

The major impetus for promoting the use of advance directives has been the Patient Self-Determination Act (PSDA) of 1990. This legislation was Congress's response to the *Cruzan* case and to the Supreme Court's subsequent recommendations. As Prendergast (2001) pointed out, the PSDA was written when it was feared that incompetent, terminally ill patients like Nancy Cruzan and Karen Quinlan were at grave risk of being treated and kept alive for unduly long periods of time, and without adequate recognition of their suffering and the suffering of their families. Advance directives were seen as a means of exercising mercy and protecting patients' autonomy by allowing them to direct treatment staff and family members in regard to their end-of-life care. It was also hoped that a discussion of values might take place at the time of completing an advance directive and that improvements in communication might therefore occur between patients, family, and staff related to issues of death and dying. As mentioned in chapter 1, there was probably also an implicit hope that there would be a resultant reduction in costly medical expenditures associated with the management of care for the terminally ill.

The PSDA required all hospitals, nursing homes, and health mainte-nance organizations that received Medicare and Medicaid funding to develop written policies on advance directives, to educate their staff about them, to inform all patients on admission to the facility or agency of their right to complete advance directives, and to supply patients with written materials about them. Every state that did not already have one subsequently passed a statute that established the legality of advance directives.

More than a decade after the enactment of the PSDA and the exten-sive promulgation of advance directives, however, many experts seem to agree that the hopes for them have yet to be realized (Prendergast, 2001; Teno, Licks, et al., 1997; Teno, Lynn, Connors, et al., 1997; Teno, Lynn, Wenger, et al., 1997; The SUPPORT Principal Investigators, 1995). Some have argued pessimistically that it always was, and remains, inevitable that this would be the case (Tonelli, 1996).

Questions About the Effectiveness of Advance Directives

Pessimism about the efficacy of advance directives has been expressed on theoretical, practical, and empirical grounds. Theoretically, Tonelli (1996) put forth the argument that the notion of projecting autonomy into the future when someone is so dramatically changed as to become nonau-tonomous may have serious problems. According to him, this extension of autonomy has been based on a theory of identity and personhood that demands a continuity of interests, values, and wishes despite profound changes in the person. As he has noted, severe illness and mounting cogni-tive deficits can change anyone's interests and values.

Whether one accepts this particular view of identity or not, Tonelli (1996) also argued, on more practical grounds, that all one needs to recog-nize is that a patient who has become mentally incapacitated may now have interests and values that have changed radically, and that have diverged from those that formed the basis for his or her advance directive. In other words, what may seem like an intolerable situation from the viewpoint of a compe-tent individual may be experienced very differently by someone whose capacity is more limited. As Dresser and Whitehouse (1994) pointed out, these patients continue to have an experiential world (albeit a changed one) from which they may derive meaning. They have suggested that the clinician's focus needs to shift away from prior preferences to the patient's current condition.

Still other potential problems with advance directives have been pointed out by Fagerlin, Ditto, Hawkins, Schneider, and Smucker (2002). These authors proposed that for advance directives, particularly living wills, to be effective, three assumptions must be met: (a) people must complete them, (b) the treatment preferences expressed in them must be authentic (i.e., they must not have changed), and (c) surrogate decision makers must be able to interpret them and make accurate predictions from them. They then reviewed the medical and psychological literature and found that the empirical evidence presents challenges for each assumption. Thus, they reported that various studies have demonstrated that disappointingly few Americans complete living wills, that substantial change and instability occur in people's treatment preferences over time, and that surrogates have considerable difficulty in predicting patients' wishes for life-sustaining treatment even when they have seen and discussed the patients' living will.

Other practical concerns have been voiced. Beauchamp and Childress (2001) noted that living wills often provide no basis for health professionals to attempt to overturn instructions that do not appear to be in the patient's best medical and palliative interests. Moreover, some patients and their surrogates do not appear to have an adequate understanding of the range of decisions that a surrogate decision maker might be called on to make, or they cannot foresee the clinical scenarios that might arise. Finally, problems with the definition of such key terms as *terminal condition* or *incurable illness* leave it open to interpretation as to when an advance directive is to take effect. If a more paternalistic practitioner took a narrow view and, for example, saw *terminal* as applying only within days or hours of death, patient autonomy could be very limited.

Probably the most troubling information about advance directives, however, has come from a large empirical investigation. The Study to Understand Prognoses and Preferences for Outcomes and Risks of Treatment (SUPPORT) was a $28 million, multisite trial of an intervention to improve advance care planning (The SUPPORT Principal Investigators, 1995). It consisted of two phases: (a) a 2-year observational study of 4,301 hospitalized patients with 1 or more of 9 life-threatening diagnoses (e.g., acute respiratory failure, metastatic colon cancer, and congestive heart failure) and (b) a 2-year intervention phase in which 4,804 patients were randomly assigned to control and intervention groups. The observation phase was intended to identify shortcomings in end-of-life care and to design an intervention to ameliorate them. In this phase, the investigators found that (a) only 47% of physicians knew when their patients preferred not to have CPR; (b) 46% of

DNR orders were not written until 2 days before death; (c) 38% of patients who died spent at least 10 days in an ICU; and (d) for 50% of conscious patients who died in the hospital, family members reported moderate to severe pain at least half the time.

In response to these findings, the investigators devised an intervention to facilitate communication between the patient and staff, and to improve decision making at the end of life. A skilled nurse facilitator was assigned to each case in the intervention group with the role of carrying out end-of-life discussions, providing the relevant health care information to patients, and convening meetings between patients, physicians, staff, and family members to discuss end-of-life issues and decisions. The nurse was free to shape her role in order to achieve the best possible communication among the concerned parties.

The investigators examined five major outcomes for the intervention: (a) the incidence and timing of DNR orders; (b) a patient–physician agreement on CPR preferences; (c) the number of days in an ICU, in a coma, or under ventilation before death; (d) the presence of pain; and (e) hospital resource use. Unfortunately, the authors found no significant difference between the intervention group and the control group in any of these outcome measures. In short, a well-designed effort to facilitate communication about end-of-life treatment choices did not seem to affect actual patient care.

In three studies that used the SUPPORT database, investigators looked more specifically at the efficacy of advance directives in regard to decision making (Teno, Licks, et al., 1997; Teno, Lynn, Connors, et al., 1997; Teno, Lynn, Wenger, et al., 1997). First, they examined the documentation of advance directives in the medical record at three different times: before the passage of the PSDA, after its passage, and after the intervention in the SUPPORT study. Teno, Lynn, Wenger et al. (1997) found that the percentage of existing advance directives was unchanged at 21% across all three groups, but the frequency of documentation in the medical record increased at each stage from 6% to 35% to 78% after the SUPPORT intervention. In spite of this improvement in documentation, it was found that only 12% of patients with advance directives had talked with a physician when completing them, and only 25% of physicians knew of their patients' advance directives. Clearly, increased documentation of advance directives did not lead to greater communication about them between patients and physicians or to greater physician awareness of them.

Second, the investigators (Teno, Licks, et al., 1997) searched for evidence that advance directives protected the expressed wishes of the patient. Most advance directives were found to either appoint a surrogate decision maker or to consist of a signed standard form. In regard to surrogate decision makers, a number of studies (e.g., Emanuel & Emanuel, 1992; Gamble, McDonald, & Lichstein, 1991) have shown that a large proportion of people who appoint a health care proxy never discuss their beliefs and desires about life-sustaining treatment with them. Other studies (e.g., Seckler, Meier, Mulvihill, & Paris, 1991; Sulmasy et al., 1998), as noted earlier, have shown proxy decision makers to be imperfect predictors of patients' wishes. Using hypothetical end-of-life scenarios on which surrogates and physicians were asked to make a substituted judgment for a patient, Seckler et al. (1991) found rates of agreement as low as 59%, while Sulmasy et al. (1998) found matching decisions in only 66% of the cases.

For those in the SUPPORT study who completed a living will, only a very few (5%) gave specific rather than pro forma instructions about life-sustaining treatment. Of those that directed forgoing treatment, the actual treatment of the patient appeared to be in conflict with the directive in slightly more than 50% of the cases. The authors concluded that current practice with advance directives yields few actual directives, and that little evidence suggested that the directives (when given) ensured an end-of-life treatment consistent with the wishes of the patient.

Finally, Teno, Lynn, Connors, et al. (1997) looked for a correlation between the documentation of advance directives and the use of hospital resources. In the SUPPORT intervention group, they found that the presence of an advance directive documented by the third hospital day was actually associated with an increase in hospital charges. Oddly, the presence of an advance directive in the control group was associated with a decrease in charges. The authors accounted for this finding by noting that far fewer advance directives (33%) were documented in the control group, and that this particular subgroup (i.e., control patients with an advance directive) was biased toward making their wishes known about less aggressive care. Whatever the case may be, no definitive evidence proved that advance directives resulted in the saving of health care resources.

Is the Problem in the Process?

Findings from the SUPPORT study seem to have offered an indictment of advance directives. Since the passage of the PSDA, advance directives have been entered into the medical record more frequently, but they have not been completed by patients more frequently. When completed, they did not seem to increase patient–physician communication about the patient's wishes. When available, they did not seem to change end-of-life care or reduce the use of hospital resources.

A notable exception to the SUPPORT findings, however, has been the experience in Oregon, which has been a leader in promoting good end-of-life care. In Oregon, it has been reported that nearly two thirds of those who die have an advance directive. Moreover, more than 90% of the families of patients with advance directives have been found to be satisfied with how their relative's end-of-life experience was managed (Wyden, 2000).

Some have argued that the fault has not been with advance directives per se, but with the process by which advance care planning has been approached (Fins, 1997). Others (e.g., Prendergast, 2001) have maintained that the negative outcome of the SUPPORT study has provided us with the raw data to try to understand why advance directives have not been more effective and how we might improve them. Both Fins (1997) and Prendergast (2001) highlighted the fact that the roles of the patient–clinician relationship and of good communication within that relationship have been largely overlooked in the standard approach to advance directives. As Fins (1997) noted, "Important life choices are not made in a formulaic or episodic manner but within the context of families and trusting relationships with clinicians" (p. 520). A checklist approach in which one answers *yes* or *no* to life support in the event of terminal illness, permanent unconsciousness, or brain damage does not seem particularly conducive to good communication and assumes that patients have preferences that can easily be determined.

Relative to the difficulties of health care proxies mentioned earlier, some evidence shows that many patients do not seem to expect their surrogates to be in perfect agreement with them on end-of-life decisions. In one study (Sehgal et al., 1992), for example, 61% of a sample of dialysis patients said that they would allow their surrogate to override their advance directive if overriding seemed to be in their best interests. The implication from this study, as well as from the review by Fagerlin et al. (2002), seemed to be that many of these patients were not hoping that their health care proxy would be someone who would rigidly follow their written directives, but someone who would be flexible, consider the patient's changing health circumstances, do their best to observe the patient's values and preferences, and decide in that context what seemed to be in the patient's best interests.

Fins (1997) criticized the investigators in the SUPPORT study for having constructed a study design that, in spite of the effort at facilitating communication, actually still made good communication difficult. As an example of the problem, he has cited how patients were asked about their preferences in terms of CPR. In effect, these seriously ill patients were asked if their heart stopped beating would they want their doctors to try to revive them (something that usually included mechanical ventilation) or not. Fins has pointed out that such a question was too narrowly cast. The patient was not given the alternative of palliative care, but rather was left with the notion that just two options were available: resuscitation or nothing. More communication about efforts to palliate or make the patient comfortable during the dying process would have seemed to be important information for patients to have when deciding about such an advance directive.

The quality of communication about advance directives is an area that has not been examined very thoroughly. Tulsky, Fischer, Rose, and Arnold (1998) attempted to explore this issue in a study in which they tape-recorded discussions about advance directives between physicians and patients. All the patients in this study had a serious medical illness, and the physicians were all experienced attending internists in an outpatient setting. The physicians were asked to give their usual discussion of advance directives to one of their individual patients. The session was taped and then coded according to certain categories for discussions of advance directives (e.g., gives rationale and elicits values).

The findings indicated that the median discussion of advance directives lasted 5.6 minutes, and physicians spoke for approximately two thirds of that time or, on average, 3.9 minutes. The patient had an average of less than 2 minutes to speak. In general, physicians seemed unlikely to attend to the emotional content of the discussion. Thus, only 29% of them acknowledged that it could be an emotionally difficult topic. Physicians in the study discussed advance directives largely by posing hypothetical scenarios, but they typically used scenarios that were relatively easy to decide. That is, they used either dire situations in which death was almost certain and most patients would reject treatment, or reversible situations in which a good chance of recovery was possible and most patients would want aggressive care. They were less likely to discuss the more commonly experienced end-of-life scenarios in which the outcome was less certain and where guidance was more frequently needed both for the physician and for the family. In addition, physicians were likely to focus on whether the patient wanted specific interventions, while not exploring the reasons for patient preferences or patient values.

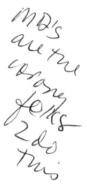

In at least one study in which an emphasis was placed on good clinician–patient communication and on a more process-oriented approach to advance care planning, the findings indicated a much more positive picture in regard to the effectiveness of advance directives. In the Lacrosse Advance Directive Study (LADS), a community-wide advance directive education program called *Respecting Your Choices* was employed (Hammes & Rooney, 1998). Remarkably, the four major health care providers in Lacrosse County, Wisconsin—an area with a population of approximately 92,000—collaborated for the purposes of the study. The education program emphasized that advance care planning was an ongoing process and shifted the focus from the completion of an advance directive document to the discussion of values and preferences. It also refocused the discussion of preferences away from autonomy toward relationships and the involvement of family and significant others. Thus, rather than asking the patient what he or she wanted, the program encouraged clinicians to ask the patient how he or she could guide loved ones to make the best decision for him or her.

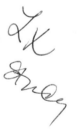

The program provided uniform training and education in the previous approach for nonphysician advance directive educators who were available and accessible at all health care organizations in the county. Patient education materials were also distributed throughout the community. The various health care organizations adopted common policies and procedures for maintaining and using advance directive documents, and documentation in the medical record was strongly encouraged.

Two years after the initiation of this program, the investigators did a retrospective study of the 540 decedents who had been under the care of the involved health care organizations (Hammes & Rooney, 1998). Although a survey done prior to the start of the program found that 15% of the population in these organizations had advance directives, it was found that 85% of the decedents had advance directives. It was also found that 95% of these advance directives were available in medical records. The decedents with advance directives had typically made their preferences known more than a year before their death (the median time was 1.2 years). Nearly all of them indicated that they were willing to limit life-sustaining treatment, and 98% actually did have some limitation of treatment. The most common rationale for forgoing life-sustaining treatment was a permanent and negative change in the quality of life. The most common preference was not to attempt CPR. When specific treatment preferences were compared with decisions made at or near the time of death, the decisions were quite consistent with the preferences stated in the advance directives. Thus, for example, 58 decedents had requested no ventilatory support. Mechanical ventilation was forgone in 17 of these cases, and in 41 cases no decision about ventilation was needed. No cases occurred in which ventilation was provided when the patient's preference had been otherwise.

The LADS study does not stand entirely alone. More recently, Molloy et al. (2000) did a randomized controlled trial with matched nursing homes in Canada. As with the LADS study, these researchers implemented a systematic and extensive educational program about advance care planning called the *Let Me Decide* program. They trained nurses as health care facilitators who then educated hospital staff, nursing home staff, residents, and families about advance directives. At any particular nursing home, a health care facilitator was required to devote 6 to 8 months of solid work just to implement the program. The Let Me Decide directive itself was far more complete than the standard advance directive in covering life-threatening illness, cardiac arrest, and feeding options for reversible and irreversible conditions. It involved a comprehensive educational process. The findings in this study were that the systematic implementation of this program reduced hospitalizations, resource use, and aggressive care for nursing home residents who did not want that level of care.

The findings in the LADS study and the study by Molloy et al. (2000) stand in marked contrast to those of the SUPPORT study. Both studies (Hammes & Rooney, 1998; Molloy et al., 2000) were limited in the sense that they assessed relatively small and homogenous samples. Moreover, the LADS study was retrospective in nature. The results of these studies, nonetheless, have suggested that if we make a strong educational effort, if we focus on meaningful discussion and communication about end-of-life issues, and if we regard advance care planning as an ongoing process rather than the completion of a form, then patients may be far more likely to understand that it can be relevant to them. If, however, advance directives are approached in a perfunctory manner and are presented by administrative clerks or hurried clinicians, then it is highly likely that we will continue to see low rates of completion and little overall impact. The PSDA has legislated the development of written policies, the distribution of written educational materials, and the provision of information about patients' rights to complete advance directives. What is more difficult to legislate, however, is the quality of communication and discussion about advance care planning.

The medical and legal language and the checklist quality of standard advance directive forms have been other factors that do not foster meaningful discussion and communication. At least two notable efforts, however, have offered alternatives to this approach. Jim Towey, founder of the non-profit organization called *Aging With Dignity* (Tallahassee, Florida), has written a combined living will and health care proxy document called *Five Wishes* (Commission on Aging with Dignity, 1998). Dr. Robert Pearlman and his colleagues at the VA Seattle Healthcare System have written a manual called *Your Life, Your Choices* on how to prepare a personalized living will (Pearlman et al., 2001). These documents are presented in ordinary language that attempts to minimize impersonal and difficult to understand medical and legal terminology. The approach in both is one that also attempts to look at not just the person's physical needs, but his or her personal, emotional, and spiritual needs as well. *Five Wishes* has been accepted as a legally valid advance directive in over 30 states. Such efforts to improve the process of completing advance directives seem encouraging.

END-OF-LIFE DECISIONS IN THE ABSENCE OF ADVANCE DIRECTIVES

As noted in the SUPPORT study cited earlier, it is estimated that only 1 in 5 people in the United States have completed a living will or named a health care proxy. Thus, in many cases, hospitals and nursing homes are faced with the dilemma of how to decide whether to discontinue treatment without any advance guidance from the patient, who is at that point unable to decide. In such cases, both the courts (e.g., *In re Quinlan*, 1976, and *Cruzan v. Director, Missouri Department of Health*, 1990) and common practice have assigned presumptive authority to the patient's closest family member as the surrogate decision maker. In terms of determining the closest family member, most health care systems have followed the order of spouse, adult child or a majority of the adult children, parents, adult siblings, adult grandchildren, or, otherwise, the nearest living relative. If no relatives are available, some systems will accept a close friend as a surrogate, provided the close friend has shown care and concern for the patient's welfare; is familiar with the patient's health, religious beliefs, and values; and is willing to provide a written statement that describes his or her relationship and familiarity with the patient.

As Beauchamp and Childress (2001) pointed out, a surrogate decision maker should have a commitment to the incompetent patient's well-being that is free of conflicts of interest. The family is presumed to be identified with the patient's interests and to have knowledge of his or her values and preferences. We know, however, that times will occur when such is not the case, and even the closest family member can have conflicts of interest. If it appears that a family member who is the designated surrogate has a serious conflict of interest or is otherwise incapable of acting as a health care proxy, the health care professionals involved have a responsibility to contest the surrogate's authority by an appeal to an independent review such as a hospital Ethics Advisory Committee (EAC) or to the courts if necessary.

More perplexing problems can occur with patients who are terminally ill, incapable of making health care decisions, and have no available surrogate. Because, in many states, the courts have not taken it upon themselves to create a pool of individuals who are readily available to act as guardians or ombudsmen, the possibility of obtaining a court-appointed surrogate often is not an easy option, except under extreme circumstances.

The institutional or hospital EAC has sometimes been asked to fill this void. The use of an EAC to advise on the treatment or nontreatment of incompetent patients remains somewhat controversial. As Kleespies, Hughes, and Gallacher (2000) noted, EACs typically consist of hospital staff who, although not part of the patient's treatment team, may identify more with the team than with the patient, and who, in any case, may find it hard to be unbiased by the needs, mores, and values of the institution for which they work. In an era when health care has been dominated by managed care and issues of cost containment, this would seem to be no small concern. As mentioned earlier, those who take on the responsibility of a surrogate should not have conflicts of interest, but rather should be partial to the interests of the patient.

These are not well-charted waters, but Beauchamp and Childress (2001) were nonetheless of the opinion that the benefits of a good EAC review may outweigh the risks. Such a review can foster open discussion and debate, and hopefully counter biased or more narrow points of view. These authors have cautioned, however, that EAC recommendations may need to be monitored and reviewed by a neutral third party such as an auditor. Checks help to ensure fair representation. In complex cases with no surrogate or where strong and unresolvable differences are held between family members of equal rank, the courts remain the last recourse. A few jurisdictions have addressed this issue proactively by assigning a particular judge to hear cases of terminally ill patients who have no available surrogate.

CONCLUSION

In this chapter, we have reviewed the ethically and legally sanctioned options available to terminally ill patients who do not want to prolong the dying process needlessly. The choices are clearly limited. When the end is near and the individual feels that little can be gained from continuing a struggle that will, in any case, have the same inevitable outcome, he or she *may be* in a position to exercise some control of how and when death will occur. If the individual is a candidate for or receives life-sustaining treatment, he or she can have it withheld or withdrawn so that the illness or condition will run its course unobstructed. If the person is in great pain, he or she could have medication increased to relieve the pain, even though it may have the effect of hastening death. If the individual is in intractable pain or is suffering unbearably, he or she might be a candidate for terminal sedation. Finally, if life is unbearable because of a terminal illness, one could voluntarily cease to eat and drink and die of dehydration. The possibility of writing a living will or of appointing a proxy decision maker continues to hold out the hope that one or the other of these options will be followed if it has been the patient's desire but he or she is no longer able to participate in the decision.

These options, however, are definitely not sufficient to make all deaths, or even most deaths, easy and comfortable. In many cases, such options simply do not apply, and even in many situations when they do, much suffering is still associated with the dying process. It is for these reasons that a significant segment of the U.S. population views assisted suicide in a favorable light, and in nations like the Netherlands voluntary euthanasia is a societally sanctioned possibility. These topics and the issues related to them are the subject matter of the next chapter.

4

THE WISH TO DIE: ASSISTED SUICIDE AND VOLUNTARY EUTHANASIA

Few patients actually die of physician-assisted suicide, even in Oregon or the Netherlands, where it is legal. Why then are the desires of this small group of patients worthy of more general concern? It is because the debate has tapped into public concern about non-physical kinds of suffering experienced by people who are dying. This small group of patients . . . can be seen as articulating a widespread public fear that the dying process represents a kind of destruction of humanness, a final indignity . . .

—Back and Pearlman, 2001, p. 344

As noted in chapter 3, our society has approved various decisions that may have the secondary effect of hastening death in terminally ill patients. Examples of such decisions would be withholding or withdrawing life-sustaining treatment, increasing analgesics and sedation to relieve suffering, terminal sedation, and so forth. These courses of action or inaction are condoned under a rationale that maintains that the primary intent is not to cause death but to relieve pain or allow the individual to control what is being done to his or her body. This rationale has been generally accepted after long debate and several watershed court decisions.

Understandably, even more controversy has surrounded proposals to legalize procedures like assisted suicide or voluntary euthanasia where clearly the primary intent is to relieve suffering by causing death. As Brody (1992) pointed out, health care professionals usually try to resolve such controversies by appeals to ethical rights and duties. Yet in the most compelling cases of intractable pain and suffering, this approach has not proven satisfactory because the ethical rights and duties on both sides have seemed so evenly balanced. Thus, one can assert a physician's basic commitment to preserve life, but in some cases, only at the cost of denying his or her duty to relieve suffering and respect autonomy.

Before considering the issues of assisted suicide and voluntary euthanasia, however, a more basic question should be asked, and that is whether or not a decision to end one's own life can ever be arrived at through a rational decision-making process and whether or not such a decision can be considered a reasonable conclusion (Kleespies, Hughes, & Gallacher, 2000; Werth, 1999a). In this chapter, we first examine the question of rational suicide and then discuss the controversy surrounding assisted suicide and voluntary euthanasia.

THE QUESTION OF RATIONAL SUICIDE

The question of whether suicide can ever be characterized as rational has been long and fiercely debated. The key arguments on both sides of this controversial topic are presented in the section below.

The Essential Arguments Pro and Con

Daniel Callahan (1999) drew attention to the fact that a distinction may be made between the *rational* and the *reasonable*. In his framework, *rational* has been taken to mean the reasoning process; that is, it refers to an orderly and consistent progression from premises to conclusions. To say that a conclusion is reasonable, however, implies not only that it was reached by a rational process but also that the premises were sound and of good quality. From this perspective, to state that an act such as suicide is rational is not to say much of importance at all. Decisions can be rational, but that does not imply they are necessarily good, bad, or reasonable. If we accept, for example, the premise that certain people are not fully human, then the decision to keep slaves might be a rational conclusion. Thus, Callahan argued that asking whether suicide is a reasonable decision is far more complex than determining whether or not it may be arrived at by a rational process.

His argument, however, was not that suicide could never be a reasonable option, but rather that, for it to be so, it would need to follow from an ideological tradition and system of values that our society does not have. He also disparaged the existing value of autonomy and self-determination as "unconscionably thin" (p. 27) as a justification for suicide. He also noted that we feel a repugnance for suicide because the individual who commits suicide has chosen to leave the human community in a way that is harmful to those of us who remain.

Although some of Callahan's arguments have logic and power, they seem deficient in several ways. First, those in our society who subscribe to the notion of rational suicide clearly see it not only as a decision resulting from a rational process of thinking but also as a potentially reasonable response to such conditions as intractable and severe pain and suffering in those who are dying (e.g., Battin, 1995; Battin, 1999; Werth, 1999a). Second, the value placed on self-determination and autonomy derives from a long and deeply held ideological tradition in the United States. It is echoed in the words of Supreme Court Justice Cardozo (cited in chapter 2) that every adult of sound mind has a right to determine what shall be done with his or her own body. This principle has been extensively applied in cases where decisions are made that hasten death, and it is not considered "thin" in these cases.

Third, proponents of rational suicide for terminally ill patients (e.g., Battin, 1994) have appealed not only to the ethical principle of autonomy but also to the principle of mercy. This viewpoint indicates that the pain and suffering of a person ought to be relieved when it is in accordance with the person's wishes and doesn't violate other moral obligations. Finally, it is not clear whether the refusal of life-sustaining treatment in the face of unbearable suffering is any less of a break in solidarity with the human community than rational suicide under the same conditions.

Opponents of rational suicide (e.g., Jay Callahan, 1999) have pointed to the fact that a majority of the large, community-based psychological autopsy studies (e.g., Chynoweth, Tonge, & Armstrong, 1980; Rich, Young, & Fowler, 1986) have found that more than 90% of adults who committed suicide suffered from a major mental or emotional disorder. The implication has been that suicide could not be the product of a rational thought process, but is almost always strongly influenced by mental illness. This traditional psychological view has held that rational suicide is a contradiction in terms because *suicide* implies an irrational act.

Jamison (1999) noted, however, that a problem exists in linking the results of psychological autopsy studies to suicide in terminally ill patients; that is, the data for such studies has usually been derived from official suicide statistics where clear evidence shows that the deaths were self-intentioned. The studies, therefore, have not taken into account secret suicides and assisted suicides that were reported as being due to natural causes. Jamison (1996), in fact, reported that he did an investigation of assisted suicides and found that the great majority of them (125 of 140) were recorded as deaths from natural causes. Moreover, in 41 of the cases, the deaths were signed off as such by the same physicians who knowingly provided the patient with the means to end his or her life. Nearly 90% of the assisted suicides in Jamison's study were never reported in the official suicide statistics.

As stated by Kleespies, Hughes, and Gallacher (2000), perhaps the most compelling argument for rational suicide comes with the patient who is terminally ill, has the capacity to make health care decisions, is suffering physically and emotionally, and may live for 6 months to a year, but wishes to die. Such a patient, when he or she is receiving life-sustaining treatment, has the legally protected right to refuse treatment and allow death to occur.

For a patient who is terminally ill and suffering, but not in need of life support systems, it is a different matter, however. If the patient has poorly controlled pain, he or she might request or agree to an increase in medication to relieve the pain. To provide relief, the medication might need to be adjusted to a point where death will be hastened in the process (the so-called double effect), yet other terminally ill patients may not have symptoms of physical pain that can be targeted easily with medication. Nonetheless, they may suffer greatly, at times immeasurably, from a series of factors, such as (a) poor health, (b) physical frailty, (c) mental confusion, (d) memory loss, (e) displacement from a home environment to a hospital or nursing home setting, (f) social death and isolation, and (g) all the personal losses that can accompany dying, millimeter by millimeter, from an extended illness. It is the public fear of this sort of suffering, which is primarily nonphysical in nature, that Back and Pearlman (2001) saw as fueling the debate over end-of-life decisions. To suggest that a competent patient who wishes to die, and is undergoing such a death, must continue to live to the bitter end because they might break solidarity with the rest of us seems insensitive to the patient's suffering.

Under such circumstances, it certainly seems conceivable that a patient might decide to end his or her life intentionally and not be considered as having impaired judgment or a mental illness. In fact, it is conceivable that such a decision might allow the individual to retain some dignity and autonomy rather than dying in an even more debilitated state. According to Werth and Cobia (1995), this appears to have been the opinion of a majority of the psychologists who participated in a survey of members of Division 29 (Psychotherapy) of the American Psychological Association (APA). Eighty-one percent of the psychologists who completed this survey (which had a 50% response rate) stated that they believed in the concept of rational suicide. The rationale most frequently given for their point of view was the existence of a hopeless condition such as a terminal illness for which there was no foreseeable improvement or relief. In a previous publication on this same topic, Werth and Liddle (1994) reported that psychotherapists viewed suicide that stemmed from a painful terminal illness as significantly more acceptable than suicide in response to such difficulties as chronic physical pain, chronic depression, or catastrophic events such as bankruptcy and so forth.

Based on the results of their survey, Werth and Cobia (1995) attempted to derive criteria for considering a suicide rational. The suggested criteria were stated as follows: (a) the person has an unremitting hopeless condition (such as a terminal illness), (b) the person makes the decision as a free choice (i.e., no coercion by others is involved), and (c) the person engages in a sound decision-making process. A sound decision-making process would include, (a) engaging in a reasoned consideration of all alternatives; (b) considering the consistency of the act with one's personal values; (c) considering the impact on significant others; (d) consulting with significant others, medical experts, and, if desired, religious advisors, and (e) having one's competence assessed by a mental health professional.

Caveats About Accepting Suicide as Rational

Despite the arguments mentioned earlier, a number of caveats should be considered before agreeing that suicide might be a reasonable decision for terminally ill patients. (It should be noted that these caveats are not unique to the rational suicide debate, but they also apply to decisions about withholding or withdrawing life-sustaining treatment [Werth, 2000].)

First, it is well known that an elevated rate of clinical depression exists among those with serious medical illnesses (Cassem, 1995). Physicians, however, who work in a medical setting and have not had psychiatric training have been found to be poor at detecting depression or judgment that may be impaired by depression (Werth et al., 2000). Block (2000) made efforts to assist physicians and other clinicians in differentiating psychological distress, grief, and depression in terminally ill patients. She has highlighted differences in symptomatology such as the unremitting nature of depression versus the fluctuating nature of grief, the anhedonia of depression versus the retention of some capacity for pleasure in those who are distressed, and so forth. Depression, of course, can influence a patient's perception to the point that a difficult situation may seem hopeless prematurely, or the benefits of continued life in terms of improving or repairing damaged relationships with family may be clouded. Even in terminally ill patients, sometimes depression can be treated and the patient's outlook may become less negative. An approach that uses supportive psychotherapy (including a life review), patient and family education, and medication (for those with severe depression) has been recommended (Block, 2000).

As Battin (1994) and Sullivan and Youngner (1994) argued, however, any evidence of depression should not necessarily be taken as indicating that the patient's decision-making capacity is impaired. Clearly, the research by Grisso and Appelbaum (1995; 1998) showed that a large percentage of depressed patients are capable of meeting even the most rigorous existing standards for decision-making capabilities.

Second, for clinicians who work with terminally ill patients and for the patients themselves, it would seem that the effort should always be to make the necessity of decisions about ending life as infrequent as possible. Good palliative care should always be practiced and should not be allowed to fall victim to the alternative of intentional death. As Kleespies and Mori (1998) noted, such an effort requires that great attention be given to pain management and comfort care, to the recognition of treatable anxiety and depression, and to assisting the patient in bringing closure to previously unresolved issues with family and friends. Attention should also be paid to supporting the patient in grieving, saying farewell, and bringing about the good death or, perhaps more realistically in Battin's terms, "the least worst death" (Battin, 1994, p. 36). In other words, the patient may miss many important end-of-life interchanges and events if he or she takes a fear-driven early exit (Block, 2001).

Third, a significant concern exists that our society could become suicide permissive. That is, if suicide is presented as a rational option in some cases (e.g., for terminally ill patients), an ideological change might occur in which suicide is seen as more socially acceptable for those in whom suicidality is a function of a treatable mental disorder rather than of a terminal illness. In fact, as discussed by Battin (1994, p. 198), there has been a "profusion of recent literary accounts favorable to suicide and assisted suicide in terminal illness cases." These accounts, as well as the previously mentioned heightened concerns about autonomy around end-of-life decisions, have already led to changing societal views of suicide.

Concern rises when one considers the possibility that the societal acceptance of suicide could influence individuals to choose suicide as an option when they otherwise would not do so. As pointed out by Hendin (1995), social acceptance alone could open the door for forms of subtle coercion in which terminally ill individuals might feel pressure to choose suicide because it is the expected or *honorable* thing to do. We would need to guard against such possibilities with appropriate ethical and professional standards that might be based on criteria such as those suggested by Werth and Cobia (1995), and/or on the issues to consider when exploring end-of-life decisions noted in Appendix F of the report by the APA Working Group (2000).

Lastly, coupled with the fear of a suicide-permissive society is the fear that elderly and terminally ill patients will be coerced into choosing suicide either by caregivers or family members. Battin (1994) provided numerous examples of situations in which an individual might feel pressured by others to end his or her life prematurely. These situations include becoming a financial burden to the family and sparing one's family members from the need to take on caretaker roles or watch the dying process. She has pointed out that families may express, in subtle and not so subtle ways, their desire to free themselves from the burden of elderly or terminally ill family members. If faced with such a scenario, does the vulnerable terminally ill person need support to resist the pressure? In addition to possible family pressures, a risk of institutional pressures is also present. Thus, if a need to cut or contain costs exists, might providers be tempted to manipulate the institutionalized elderly

Permissive attit

Elderly coerced

or terminally ill person to choose suicide? Again, it would be necessary to guard against such eventualities with a vigilant approach to professional and organizational standards.

THE QUESTION OF ASSISTED SUICIDE

Whether the suicide of a terminally ill person could be a rational or reasonable decision that might preserve some dignity and autonomy for the individual is one question. Whether such a death should be assisted by a second party is another. Clearly, some terminally ill patients are capable of ending their own lives should they wish to do so, but others may be too physically debilitated or restricted by their situation to have such an option. At times, they ask others, often their doctors, to assist them. Assisted suicide has been defined as the practice of providing a competent patient with a prescription for medication to be used with the primary intention of ending his or her own life (Meier et al., 1998). What gives rise to such a patient request?

It is known from the experience with assisted death in the Netherlands that physical pain is usually not the driving force (van der Maas, van Delden, Pijnenborg, & Looman, 1991). Rather, loss of dignity, feelings of dependency, and poor quality of life have been reported as major reasons. In the United States, Breitbart, Rosenfeld, and Passik (1996) surveyed a large sample of HIV-infected patients about their attitudes toward physician-assisted suicide. They also examined the relationship between interest in physician-assisted suicide and physical and psychosocial variables. Of the patients in this sample, 63% supported policies favoring physician-assisted suicide, and 55% acknowledged considering it as an option for themselves. Psychological distress and social factors were much stronger predictors of interest in physician-assisted suicide than pain or other physical symptoms. Moreover, although depression was a major element in predicting interest in physician-assisted suicide, it was by no means the sole determinant. Thus, factors such as the experience of the painful death of a friend or family member and increasing social isolation were also major determinants.

Recently, a group of investigators (Lavery, Boyle, Dickens, Maclean, and & Singer, 2001) attempted to collect data on the reasons for requesting physician-assisted suicide by interviewing patients who had actually considered pursuing assisted suicide or euthanasia. They did a qualitative study of 32 people who were HIV positive or had AIDS. Of this group, 63% had actually decided to seek either assisted suicide or euthanasia, 28% were still undecided, and 9% had decided to reject the idea. The investigators did face-to-face interviews with the participants. They used open-ended questions to pursue five themes: autonomy, dignity, suffering, the role of others, and end-of-life care. They then analyzed the responses and felt that they could categorize them into two main factors associated with requests for assisted suicide or euthanasia: (a) fear of disintegration and (b) loss of community.

For Lavery et al. (2001), fear of disintegration seemed to refer to the progressive loss of function associated with advancing AIDS. As one participant in their study put it,

AIDS related

> "You've become a sack of potatoes to be moved from spot to spot, to be rushed back and forth from the hospital, to be carried to your doctors' appointments or wheeled in a wheelchair, and it really does take away any self-worth, any dignity, or any will to continue to live." (p. 365)

Loss of community, on the other hand, seemed to refer to the progressive decline of desire and opportunity to initiate and maintain close personal relationships because of loss of mobility and alienation from others, that is, experiencing the social death and isolation mentioned earlier.

The study by Lavery et al. was very limited in that it was strictly qualitative. No effort was made to validate the constructs that were derived, the sample size was very small, and the sample was restricted to HIV/AIDS patients. The findings must be regarded as only suggestive, but they are consistent with other observations of terminally ill patients who requested assisted death in Oregon (Hedberg, Hopkins, & Southwick, 2002; Sullivan, Hedberg, & Hopkins, 2001), in Washington (Back, Wallace, Starks, & Pearlman, 1996), and in the Netherlands (van der Maas et al., 1991). They suggest that a strong psychological or emotional component is part of the suffering that drives patients to request aid in dying. It is the sort of suffering that is not addressed by the management of physical pain, and for which palliative care, as well as psychological or psychiatric interventions, may not be entirely effective. It has affected a larger proportion of the terminally ill population in developed countries because of the new epidemiological pattern of death from degenerative diseases discussed in chapter 1.

Until approximately 3 decades ago, the norm was for the terminally ill person to attempt to live and fight off death, regardless of the misery involved, for as long as possible. Our society now seems to be reconsidering these presumably heroic efforts and has given approval to such decisions as withholding or withdrawing life-sustaining treatment when it is considered pointless to go on. According to Brody (1992), modern medicine has tacitly encouraged the approach of fighting death until the last breath because medical treatment providers have been inclined to view a patient's death as a failure or, when death has seemed inevitable, they have seen the dying process as reason to disengage from the patient. As a result, patients have been left with the fear that physicians will either overtreat them with high-tech interventions or abandon them to suffering. It is in this context that the debate over assisted suicide has arisen.

The Essential Arguments Pro and Con

The essential arguments for and against assisted suicide have been succinctly outlined by Battin (1995). Those in favor have argued primarily on the basis of the ethical principles of autonomy and mercy, as mentioned earlier in this chapter. The argument on the basis of autonomy is that the individual has the right to determine, as much as possible, the course of his or her own life. Dying is a part of the life course, and the individual also has the right to determine, as much as possible, the course and conditions of his or her own dying. Some may object that a truly autonomous choice is rarely possible because, in terminal illness, depression and other emotional disturbances are likely to be factors that influence decisions. However, as presented in chapter 2, depression and even other major mental illness, such as schizophrenia, do not necessarily preclude competent decision making. MÆ

The argument on the basis of mercy is that no one should have to endure pointless suffering when he or she is dying. If the physician cannot relieve the patient's suffering by other means and the patient wishes to die to end his or her agony, the physician should assist the individual in ending his or her life in the most comfortable way. Although advances have been made in pain management and palliative care, clearly we have not eliminated all pain, and we certainly have not eliminated the psychological suffering noted in the study by Lavery et al. (2001). Of course, the option exists of attempting to address such intractable pain and suffering with complete sedation, but proponents of assisted suicide have argued that this is tantamount to causing death. Finally, those opposed to assisted death have noted that instances of transformation and growth have emerged from prolonged suffering at the end of life (Block, 2001), yet it is not clear how often and for whom this occurs.

Opponents of assisted suicide have primarily argued (a) that killing is intrinsically wrong, (b) that it puts us on the slippery slope where it will be too easy to engage in the killing of vulnerable people who do not wish to die, and (c) that the physician's traditional role as a beneficent healer would be compromised if he or she entered into actively assisting in bringing about death. Those who have put forth the first of these arguments believe that the taking of a human life is morally unacceptable. In cases where it is socially condoned (e.g., in war or with capital punishment), it is seen as justified by self-defense or by the guilt of the individual killed. Proponents of assisted suicide, however, have argued that if it is acceptable to take a life under these circumstances, then it should also be acceptable when it is the choice of a competent person to die.

Those who have been concerned about the slippery slope, so to speak, feel that cost pressures and factors like insensitivity and the tendency to follow the easiest course will put physicians and institutions at risk of promoting assisted death in cases where it would not be justified. Thus, for example, patients who have suffered serious brain damage and might be considered by some to be social and familial burdens could be at risk of having surrogates make decisions that favor requests for assisted death when hope for improvement is still present. The question for proponents of assisted suicide is whether it is possible to develop effective protections against such abuses. In this regard, Orentlicher (2000) noted that all the slippery slope arguments for prohibiting assisted suicide are arguments that apply equally well to the withdrawal or withholding of life-sustaining treatment where significant potential for abuse also exists. Medical ethicists seem to feel, however, that we have been able to develop and maintain adequate safeguards in allowing competent patients to refuse treatment at the end of life (Beauchamp & Childress, 2001). Would this not seem to indicate that assisted suicide could also be regulated to protect against abuses?

slippery slope

In terms of the physician's role, the argument has been that permitting physicians to be involved in killing is a violation of the ethical principles of beneficence and nonmaleficence, and will undermine patients' trust in them as healers. Proponents of assisted suicide have countered by pointing out, again, that a physician's actions in withdrawing or withholding treatment are just as deliberate as in assisted suicide, and that it is inconsistent to apply the beneficence and *do-no-harm* principles only to assisted dying (Jamison, 1997). Moreover, they have argued that patients will trust their physicians more if they know that they will not abandon them when they are suffering gravely and alternative efforts at relief have failed.

Emanuel, Fairclough, Daniels, and Claridge (1996) gathered data relative to this argument. In a survey of oncology patients and oncologists, they found that 53% of oncologists, but only 37.2% of cancer patients, thought that discussions between patients and physicians on end-of-life care that included mention of euthanasia or physician-assisted suicide would reduce patients' trust in the physician. By way of contrast, 41.6% of patients, but only 15.6% of oncologists, thought that such discussions would increase patients' trust in the physician. Although further study is needed, the disparity between physicians and patients on this issue suggests that physicians could be somewhat overconcerned about a loss of the patient's trust as an outcome. Emanuel et al. (1996), however, pointed out that depressed patients in their study were more likely than nondepressed patients, and patients with physical pain, to trust their physicians after discussions of physician-assisted suicide. This finding raises the question of the degree to which patient interest in such discussions may be driven by depression and might be decreased if depression were relieved.

MDD

The Polarities of Assisted Suicide: Dr. Kevorkian and Dr. Quill

In June 1990, Janet Adkins, a 54-year-old grandmother from Oregon who was in the early stages of Alzheimer's disease, had Dr. Jack Kevorkian attach her to his "suicide machine" while she lay on a cot in the rear of a

Volkswagen van. He inserted an intravenous line in her arm and started a saline solution flowing. The machine was constructed so that Mrs. Adkins could press a button to inject first a sedative (thiopental) and then potassium chloride, which would cause her heart to stop beating. She pressed the button and became the first of Dr. Kevorkian's assisted suicides (Battin, 1995; Beauchamp & Childress, 2001). Until he was convicted of second-degree murder in 1999, Dr. Kevorkian is known to have assisted in the deaths of 93 people, and this may be a conservative estimate because allegedly a number of assisted deaths took place that he did not make public (Canetto & Hollenshead, 1999).

It is noteworthy that Dr. Kevorkian's first assisted suicide was someone who was not terminally ill. Mrs. Adkins was in the early stages of Alzheimer's disease, and she was reportedly still capable of enjoying activities with her husband and playing tennis with her son. She might have had several more years of active life before she went into a more serious decline. She believed that she was slowly deteriorating, and she did not want to suffer the mental confusion, loss of memory, and loss of ability to recognize her own family that was likely to ensue. She apparently had discussions about her concerns with her family, her minister, and her local doctor over the period of a year. Her family supported her wish to seek an assisted death. Her meetings with Dr. Kevorkian, however, consisted of a few brief discussions over a weekend followed by her use of the suicide machine. Dr. Kevorkian was not her treating physician. He did not examine her to attempt to confirm her diagnosis or to establish her decision-making capacity for making such a profound decision. He did not have a mental health background that might allow him to evaluate her emotional state or stability.

Janet Adkins was not the only one of Dr. Kevorkian's cases where such circumstances prevailed. Canetto and Hollenshead (1999) reviewed 75 of the Kevorkian cases (from 1990 to 1997) and found that 69% of them had illnesses that were not in the terminal phase. Rather, chronic but debilitating illnesses such as multiple sclerosis (25% of cases) and amyotrophic lateral sclerosis (15% of cases) were the most prevalent diagnoses. (This profile can be contrasted with that in Oregon and in the Netherlands where 72% and 80% of the respective assisted deaths have been people with a diagnosis of terminal cancer [Roscoe, Malphurs, Dragovic, & Cohen, 2001].) The medical examiner in the Kevorkian cases actually found no evidence of physical disease in five cases. Four of these five had a history of depression, and most of them had a history of serious personal problems, such as having been victims of abuse.

Nearly 70% of Kevorkian's assisted suicide cases were women of European American descent. Given that, in the general population, women are less likely than men to commit suicide by a ratio of 1:4, this finding led Canetto and Hollenshead (1999) to speculate about the gender psychology that may have been operative in the Kevorkian cases. For example, women who are disabled might be more likely to have devalued lives and therefore be more inclined to seek a hastened death, or women who are suicidal might seek assisted death because they prefer not to die alone.

Clearly, the methods of Dr. Kevorkian can be questioned for many reasons. He had an alarmingly superficial knowledge of the medical and psychological condition of his clients. Although he is said to have recommended that all candidates for assisted suicide be examined first by a psychiatrist, he apparently violated this guideline repeatedly (Canetto & Hollenshead, 1999). He had no long-standing clinician–patient relationship that might have permitted him to explore possible alternate solutions. His practices were obviously very different than the standard practices in the state of Oregon where physician-assisted suicide has been legalized. He stands as an example of how the right to die movement can go awry because of a lack of accountability and regulation. The fact that so many people sought his assistance in dying, however, has also pointed to the inadequacies in our medical and social institutions for alleviating the suffering of those with chronic, debilitating illnesses.

Although Dr. Kevorkian has been imprisoned, it has not meant an end to the apparent demand (among a certain segment of the population) for *deliverance* from the agonies of some debilitating or terminal illnesses. Thus, Ogden (2001) reported on the rise of the *NuTech* movement, a group of right to die activists who are more covert than Dr. Kevorkian and who advocate non-physician-assisted suicide via technological devices that leave little evidence of their use. These devices include systems for breathing inert gases as well as a closed-circuit breathing system that quickly reduces what is circulated through the system to recycled nitrogen (resulting in death by hypoxia). As Ogden has pointed out, the emphasis on the use of technology in this movement seems to depersonalize the dying process. Moreover, no physician or regulatory oversight is set up to ensure mental competence, informed consent, and the exploration of palliative options.

In marked contrast to the assisted suicides of Dr. Kevorkian and the NuTech movement is a case described by Dr. Timothy Quill (1991). Diane was a 45-year-old woman for whom Dr. Quill had been a treatment provider for 8 years. Toward the end of this time, she developed acute myelomonocytic leukemia, a disease with a survival rate of 25% with treatment, but certain death in months or possibly weeks without treatment. Treatment would have consisted of induction chemotherapy followed by consolidation chemotherapy followed by bone marrow transplantation. Such treatments are difficult to tolerate and result in weeks and months of hospitalization with nausea, vomiting, hair loss, and probable infectious complications. Diane wanted nothing to do with this. She shared with Dr. Quill that she feared that she would die during treatment (as the majority of patients did) and that she would suffer terribly from the side effects of chemotherapy and from loss of function and control of her body. Although he offered support and palliation, Dr. Quill could not say that her fears would not be realized. In fact, he noted in his account of the case that the last four patients in his hospital with the same disease had died very painful deaths during treatment.

Since the time in which an effective treatment could be initiated was limited, Dr. Quill met with Diane several times in the space of a week. He obtained a second hematology consultation. He and his patient discussed in detail the meaning and implications of treatment and nontreatment. Diane also discussed her thoughts and feelings with a psychologist whom she had seen in the past. Ultimately, her family and Dr. Quill supported her decision to refuse treatment and arrangements were made for home hospice care.

Diane, however, was a person for whom it was very important to main- tain control and to die in a dignified manner. Although Dr. Quill explained the philosophy of comfort care to her, she had seen people suffer through what was considered comfort and she did not find it acceptable. When the time came, she wanted to end her life without great suffering. With further discussion, Dr. Quill became convinced that Diane was so concerned about dying a lingering death that her preoccupation with it would interfere with her ability to get the most out of her remaining time with friends and family. He informed her that the Hemlock Society might have information helpful to her.

A week later, Diane contacted Dr. Quill with a request for barbiturates for sleep. They had a lengthy discussion. Although she was indeed having trouble sleeping, it also seemed evident to Dr. Quill that she wanted the option of ending her life and that it would free her from her fears about the manner of her death. He also found that she was not despondent and that she was making deep and meaningful connections with her family and friends. He gave her a prescription for a barbiturate and made sure that she knew how to use it for sleep and also the amount that would be needed in order to com- mit suicide. They agreed to meet regularly, and certainly before she would take her own life.

Diane then spent several very intense months with her family. Her son stayed home from college and her husband was able to do his work at home so that the family could be together. She also visited with her closest friends. Eventually, bone pain, weakness, fatigue, and fevers worsened and began to dominate her life. Dr. Quill, her family, and the hospice workers did their utmost to reduce her suffering and provide comfort, but it became clear that her limited future held only those things that she had most dreaded, that is, increased suffering, dependence on others, and choices between pain and sedation. At this point, Diane called her closest friends and had them come to see her for a final goodbye. She also had a final meeting and a farewell with Dr. Quill.

On the day of her death, Diane said goodbye to her husband and son and asked them to leave her alone for an hour. They honored her request and subsequently found her lying on the couch. She reportedly seemed at peace

"Self" Control is a Major Issue

with no sign of struggle or distress. Her husband and son called Dr. Quill who came to the home and pronounced her dead. The family seemed to have no doubts about how she had chosen to die. By his report, Dr. Quill then called the medical examiner and informed him that a hospice patient had died of acute leukemia. He attributed her death to her disease rather than to suicide to avoid possible criminal prosecution for himself and her family, and, as he noted, "to continue to shield society from the knowledge of the degree of suffering that people often undergo in the process of dying" (Quill, 1991, p. 694).

The differences between the assisted suicides of Janet Adkins and Diane seem evident. Janet Adkins died in the back of a van far from home with the assistance of a physician (Kevorkian) who knew little about her or her condition. She was not terminally ill and might have been able to have several more years of meaningful life. Diane died in her home with the assistance of a physician (Quill) who knew her well and after lengthy discussions with her doctor and her family. She was terminally ill and suffering from her illness. Her options for relief had been thoroughly explored.

Dr. Quill could be criticized on the grounds that he potentially broke a New York State law against assisted suicide and lied to the medical examiner about the cause of death. It might also be argued that he violated the ethical principles of beneficence and nonmaleficence by his participation in causing a patient's death. Ethicists like Beauchamp and Childress (2001), however, have argued that Dr. Quill respected the autonomy of a competent patient and was guided by mercy in allowing her to avoid further suffering and the dehumanizing aspects of a lingering and painful death. If he dissembled to the medical examiner, he may have compensated by speaking openly to the entire health care community. Moreover, many would argue that assisting a terminally ill patient with the best option for relief from his or her suffering does not constitute a violation of beneficence and nonmaleficence.

The Distinction Between a Justified Act and a Legitimized Practice

Religious beliefs and convictions aside, it could be argued that Dr. Quill was not unethical or immoral in assisting Diane with her suicide. Depending on one's perspective, his particular act might well be construed as justifiable under the circumstances. It is perhaps most remarkable in that Dr. Quill published an account of it, while other physicians have done similar things for ages, but in the shadows of medical practice.

At least three surveys speak to this issue. Back et al. (1996) did an anonymous survey of physicians in the state of Washington and found that 26% of them had been asked at least once to provide assistance with suicide. These physicians reported writing a prescription to be used for suicide in 24% of the cases where it was requested. In a national survey of physicians in the 10 specialities where they are most likely to receive requests for aid in dying,

Meier et al. (1998) found that 18.3% of the respondents had received at least one request for medication to be used for suicide. In cases where it was requested, 16% of the physicians said that they had written a prescription for a lethal dose of medication. Finally, Slome, Mitchell, Charlebois, Benevedes, and Abrams (1997) did a survey of physicians in an association dedicated to providing health care to patients who are HIV infected. They found that 53% of the physicians who participated in the study (N = 118) had prescribed, on at least one occasion, a lethal amount of medication at a patient's request. The mean number of such prescriptions per provider was 4.2. Given such findings, Dr. Quill's actions with Diane do not seem so extreme. In fact, the majority of voters in one state (Oregon) would undoubtedly concur with Dr. Quill's assistance in this case.

Perspectives on Assisted Suicide in Oregon

The 1994 voter-approved Oregon Death with Dignity Act (ODDA) permits physicians to prescribe a lethal amount of medication that can be used to hasten death for competent, terminally ill persons who voluntarily request it. In a survey of the attitudes of Oregon psychologists toward physician-assisted suicide and the ODDA, Fenn and Ganzini (1999) found that 91% of the respondents felt that for a competent terminally ill person both suicide and assisted suicide were acceptable morally as either a matter of individual choice or at least under certain conditions. When those surveyed were asked if a physician should be allowed to write a prescription whose sole purpose would be to allow such a patient to end his or her life, 85% responded either *always* (29%) or *under some circumstances* (56%). Eighty-two percent of the psychologists indicated that they would consider obtaining a physician's assistance to end their own lives *under some circumstances*, and the most commonly given circumstance had to do with alleviating pain and suffering (74%). Thus, the results of this survey indicated that the majority of psychologists in Oregon appeared to believe in the application of the principle of mercy and the relief of suffering for terminally ill patients under certain conditions, even when that relief entailed assistance in suicide by another party (i.e., a physician). The extent to which these results can be generalized to psychologists in other regions of the United States has not been tested empirically.

The actual experience with assisted suicide in Oregon is limited because it has been legalized for a relatively brief period of time. (The ODDA was enacted in October 1997.) At the time of this writing, studies of the first 4 years in which assisted suicide was legal have been published (Chin, Hedberg, Higginson, & Fleming, 1999; Hedberg, Hopkins, & Southwick, 2002; Sullivan, Hedberg, & Fleming, 2000; Sullivan, Hedberg, & Hopkins, 2001). In the first year, 16 people who had received prescriptions for lethal medication used them and died, while in the second, third, and fourth years, 27, 27, and 21 people respectively did so. Of this total of 91 people who died by assisted suicide over a 4-year period, 44 were male and 47 were female. All but three were of European American descent. Twenty-three had been referred for a mental health evaluation prior to receiving the prescription. In the first year, the 16 assisted suicides constituted 6 out of every 10,000 deaths in Oregon, while in the second and third years, the assisted suicides accounted for 9 out of every 10,000 deaths and in the fourth year 7 out of every 10,000 deaths. The primary factors cited by physicians for the requests for assisted death were loss of autonomy, loss of control of one's bodily functions, and the inability to participate in activities that made life enjoyable. Neither pain nor financial concerns were cited as major factors.

These findings have been interpreted quite differently by proponents and opponents of assisted suicide, and the reports themselves have been criticized on methodological grounds. Proponents have seen the results as evidence that the value placed on autonomy in the United States is a strong motive for seeking assisted suicide, while opponents have argued that if these particular patients had received better psychosocial support and comfort care, they would not have sought assisted death. Proponents felt that the complaints about poor physical functioning demonstrated the value placed on independence and control. Opponents stated that these patients may have been reacting to the stigma placed on physical disabilities, and that, with more time and better services, they might have felt like living for a longer period.

Foley and Hendin (1999) criticized the Oregon report. These authors noted that it relied solely on information obtained from physicians, with no data directly from the individuals who actually sought assisted suicide. Moreover, they contended that because the ODDA does not require a psychiatric evaluation for patients seeking assisted suicide, the report could not give accurate data on the degree to which depression might have been impairing the judgment of those making requests. They also argued that the report provided no data on how thoroughly physicians assessed the reasons for patients' requests for aid in dying or on how adequately they had addressed palliative and hospice care options for these patients.

Coombs, Lee, and Werth (2000) began to gather information that might eventually address Foley and Hendin's initial criticism. Using data collected from those who contacted the organization *Compassion in Dying* about using the ODDA, they have presented first-hand reports from 10 individuals who died in the first year of ODDA using medication prescribed under the Act. The individuals involved were asked to examine a list of elements of suffering that Compassion in Dying provides and to identify those factors that would determine a choice of assisted death for them. The majority of responses (from those who made such a choice) had to do with the loss of general control and the loss of control over bodily functions. The 10 patients died relatively comfortably. After taking the medication, they fell into, and remained in, a coma within 1 to 10 minutes. Because they took an antiemetic first, no vomiting or aspiration occurred. The time until death ranged from 10 minutes to 11 and a half hours, with most occurring within 50 minutes. All 10 of these patients took the medication in their home. In each case, a combination of family members, physicians, clergy, compassion volunteers, or hospice staff was present. As the authors noted, no patient died alone.

Although they did not gather data directly from those who actually sought assisted death, Ganzini et al. (2000) recently presented findings that are relevant to the last two of Foley and Hendin's criticisms. In a survey of Oregon physicians who were eligible to prescribe lethal medications under ODDA, they identified 144 who had received requests for lethal prescriptions. These physicians reported symptoms and values that had played an important part in the patient's decision to request assisted death. The most frequently reported reasons had to do with loss of independence, poor quality of life, feeling ready to die, wanting to control the circumstances of their own death, and physical pain. It was, in fact, said to be uncommon for patients to cite reasons such as feeling they were a burden to others or that they lacked social support. Eighty-one percent of the patients who actually died by assisted suicide were enrolled in a hospice program at the time of death. Physicians attempted interventions such as pain and symptom control, referral to a hospice or palliative care program, a mental health consultation, a trial on antidepressant or antianxiety medication, and so forth, with 142 of the 144 patients who requested a lethal prescription. In 42 cases, one or more interventions resulted in the patient changing his or her mind about wanting assisted suicide.

Despite the promising findings reported by Coombs, Lee, and Werth (2000) and Ganzini et al. (2000), there may be good reason to be cautious about more widespread legalization of physician-assisted suicide in the United States at this time. On the one hand, the state of Oregon has developed a health care infrastructure (including a strong commitment to pain management and workable relationships with local hospice programs) (Jackson, 2000; Wyden, 2000) that could support the ODDA and might not exist in other states. On the other hand, the criticisms of the Oregon report noted earlier have not been fully answered, and the same can be said for the widely varying accounts of assisted suicide and voluntary euthanasia in the Netherlands where they have been practiced for some time.

The Relevance of the Experience in the Netherlands for the U.S.

Utilizing essentially the same database, some have argued that the Dutch have lost adherence to medical standards and have abandoned efforts at palliative care to the convenience of euthanasia or assisted suicide as the solution for those who are terminally ill (Hendin, 1999). Others have maintained that the results of two carefully conducted nationwide studies of euthanasia and assisted suicide that were commissioned by the Dutch government (van der Maas et al., 1996) can hardly be construed as indicating that the Netherlands has begun a "descent into depravity" (Angell, 1996, p. 1677). Rather, the studies found that only a small percentage of deaths in the Netherlands (2–3%) were as a result of euthanasia or assisted suicide. Given such differences in interpretation, however, it would seem wise to continue to study developments in regard to assisted death in the Netherlands and in Oregon before advocating more universal legalization.

In addition, although the slippery slope argument is disparaged by some for its lack of empirical support, it may be of more concern in a country like the United States than in the Netherlands. If restraints against causing death are removed in our country, social forces may make it more difficult to prevent abuse. Thus, the health care system in the United States has continued to be preoccupied with managing care and medical cost containment, a situation that could easily lead to callous and coercive practices concerning suicide and terminally ill patients. Although assisted death might be an option that is seldom abused in a country like the Netherlands that has universal health coverage, it could be far more problematic in the United States. Here literally millions of impoverished and vulnerable people are without adequate coverage and could feel pressure from families, health care institutions, and society in general to accept cost-saving solutions when seriously ill. In addition, one needs to think of groups such as the increasing number of elderly persons with serious and costly medical problems and how they might be placed at risk by mounting social pressure to contain expenditures. Our country, in fact, might be better served if it focused on attaining a more stable health care environment where resources are more readily available to all before considering the legalization of assisted suicide.

more reasonable [handwritten marginal note]

The author is in agreement with Beauchamp and Childress (2001) who maintained that justifying a particular act such as Dr. Quill's assistance in the suicide of Diane is distinct from justifying a practice or public policy that legitimates the regular performance of such an act. As they have noted, a rule of practice or a policy that prohibits assistance in dying may be justified, even if it excludes some acts of assisted death that in themselves are morally justified. The problem is that the legalization of assisted death runs very serious risks of abuse (as mentioned above) and, on balance, could cause more harm than benefit. Such concerns may have, in part, motivated the Dutch, who for years condoned assisted death on an individual basis but refused to legalize it. Thus, assisted death in the Netherlands remained illegal by statute and a crime, but was seen as legally defensible under a plea of *force majeure* and if it met a set of guidelines promulgated by the Royal Dutch Medical Association. *Force majeure* in the Dutch legal system is a plea based on a conflict between a physician's duty to obey the law and his or her duty to obey the demands of medical ethics and the wishes of his or her patient (Battin, 1994). If they conscientiously observed these guidelines with terminal patients who had exhausted other alternatives for the relief of suffering, Dutch physicians could be relatively sure they would not be prosecuted.

An analogous understanding with the legal system might be helpful in the United States in that it would seem to convey a message that discourages abuse, but also informs patients that if they are dying and in unrelieved misery, they need not be abandoned and forced to endure great suffering when they feel that nothing can be gained from doing so. Yet as Kamisar (1998) pointed out, dangers also exist in attempting to achieve such a *middle ground*. From a legal perspective, if exceptions are made, it can erode public confidence in the administration of our laws and communicate approval or authorization for physician-assisted suicide more broadly, the very thing that it was hoped could be avoided. Kamisar, however, has no immediate way out of this dilemma and concludes that "Sometimes, I am afraid, what appear to be agonizingly subtle and complex problems turn out to be just that" (p. 1146).

Until the Dutch recently legalized assisted death, the system of keeping it formally illegal but justifiable in cases of exceptional suffering seemed to work for them, and there may, in fact, be some basis for thinking that such an agreement might be feasible in particular states or jurisdictions in this country. In a national survey of prosecuting attorneys, Meisel, Jernigan, and Youngner (1999) presented the participants with four end-of-life scenarios that ranged from withdrawing nutrition and hydration to providing morphine tablets for suicide to a terminally ill patient with a brain tumor. The findings suggested considerable willingness among the attorneys to tolerate physician-assisted suicide even though it is formally a crime. Thus, 60% of the respondents felt that times can occur when physician-assisted suicide may be morally justified, and 78.8% said that, if they were in the same position as the patient with the brain tumor, they would want their own request for pills to commit suicide to be honored. Sixty percent said that they would not take measures that might lead to prosecution if death ensued from the assisted suicide of a terminally ill patient.

Proposed Criteria for Justified Assisted Suicide

Given that some acts of assisted suicide could seemingly be justified, one must ask, under what conditions or by what criteria would this be so? In this regard, it is instructive to consider two sets of proposed criteria (i.e., those by Quill, Cassel, & Meier [1992] and those by Beauchamp & Childress [2001]) as well as the ODDA. In reviewing the criteria of Quill et al. and Beauchamp and Childress, it is apparent that the two criteria have considerable overlap. The points that they have in common are as follows:

- The individual has incurable, unremitting, and unacceptable suffering.
- The individual's request to die is made voluntarily and on his or her own initiative.

- The request to die is made repeatedly or is durable.
- The individual is considered competent to make a decision, or his or her judgment is not distorted.
- A meaningful doctor–patient relationship exists.
- Consultation with another physician or physicians is made.

In addition to these shared criteria, Beauchamp and Childress (2001) also emphasized the need for a decision-making process that is not only voluntary and engaged in by a competent person but one that is also informed and involves a consideration and rejection of alternate courses of action. They have stressed that this decision making would best be done in a supportive but critical and probing environment. They recommended the use of means for suicide that are as painless and comfortable as possible.

Quill et al. (1992), on the other hand, indicated that one must be sure that the decision for assisted suicide is not the result of inadequate comfort care. They have suggested that, at the individual's discretion, his or her family might be informed of the decision-making process and spiritual counseling might be offered. Werth and Cobia (1995), who proposed criteria for rational suicide (not necessarily assisted suicide), might add that the congruence of the act with one's values should be considered, along with the impact of such an act on the individual's significant others.

The ODDA, of course, also has conditions for assisted suicide. It applies to citizens of Oregon who are considered terminally ill or, according to their definition, those who are expected to die within 6 months. The patient's primary physician and a consultant are required to confirm the diagnosis and prognosis, and determine the patient's decision-making capacity or competence. If either believes that the patient's judgment is impaired by depression or another psychological or psychiatric disorder, they are to refer the patient to counseling. For more detailed direction in assessing mental capacity, Werth, Benjamin, and Farrenkopf (2002) proposed a relatively extensive set of guidelines which they developed to be specifically applicable to the ODDA.

The ODDA, similar to Quill et al. and Beauchamp and Childress, requires voluntariness and durability of the request. Thus, the patient must make 1 written and 2 oral requests to his or her physician, and the 2 oral requests must be separated by at least 15 days. Physicians must report all prescriptions that they write for lethal medications to the Oregon Health Division (ODDA, 1995).

It is noteworthy that Quill et al. (1992) did not limit the application of their criteria to terminally ill patients. They stated that they "do not want to exclude arbitrarily persons with incurable, but not imminently terminal, progressive illnesses, such as amyotrophic lateral sclerosis or multiple sclerosis" (p. 1381). They seemed to have a strong emphasis on the principle of mercy and on an option for the relief of unrelenting and intolerable suffering, regardless of whether the patient is imminently terminal. The ODDA, on the other hand, is limited to terminally ill people, and Orentlicher (2000) argued that that is an important safeguard against abuse. In support of his position, he has noted that, because Dr. Kevorkian did not limit his services to terminally ill patients, he is presumed to have assisted in the deaths of some who did not suffer from serious and irreversible illness, but rather from despondency that may have been alleviated. Orentlicher's point is that with terminal illness as a criterion for assisted suicide, it is far more likely that a choice to die will reflect "a rational trade-off between quality of life and length of life than when a person is not terminally ill" (p. 499).

Although the ODDA and Orentlicher seem to have taken the more conservative, safer, and more easily defined course, it is important to remember that prognostications about time until death are very inexact, and the presumed clarity of definition (i.e., 6 months or less to live) may be questionable. Moreover, Foley and Hendin (1999) suggested that such a limited requirement (terminal illness) fails to encourage physicians to inquire into the physical and emotional suffering that might underlie a request for assisted death, and, of course, such an inquiry might lead to alternative solutions.

Obviously, the issue of criteria for what may seem to be justified assisted suicide is far from settled and will need to be debated and refined for some time to come. Any physician who might be confronted with a potentially justifiable request for aid in dying would need to consider the criteria that have been proposed in the literature and decide on an individual basis which solution might work best for the patient and for him- or herself. As Jamison (1997) suggested, "assisted death should be considered an extraordinary event—one that is made available, with hesitation, to a restricted group of patients who are suffering intolerably despite the provision of the highest quality of care" (p. 8).

THE QUESTION OF VOLUNTARY EUTHANASIA

Voluntary euthanasia has been defined as the practice of injecting a patient with a lethal dose of medication, with the primary intention of ending the patient's life (Meier et al., 1998). Although euthanasia has been the preferred form of assisted death in the Netherlands, proponents in the United States have seemed more comfortable with physician-assisted suicide (Jamison, 1997). In this regard, it is noteworthy that the state of Washington's Initiative 119 and California's Proposition 161, both of which would have legalized physician-performed euthanasia and physician-assisted suicide, were defeated at the polls in the early 1990s. The ODDA, however, which only legalized physician-assisted suicide, passed on two occasions, initially in 1994 and again in 1997 when the Oregon legislature placed a measure on the ballot to repeal the Act (Coombs, Lee, and Werth, 2000). Some have argued that this preference reflects American discomfort with having physicians directly involved in causing death as well as a prevailing opinion that authorizing voluntary euthanasia invites greater risk (than assisted suicide) of a societal slide down the slippery slope that could lead to nonvoluntary and involuntary euthanasia.

Brody (1992) noted that physician-performed voluntary euthanasia should not be discounted on the grounds that the physician is too involved as a causal agent of death. Such a position could also be construed as abandoning the patient in a time of great need and abrogating one's responsibility to relieve suffering. Rather, he has presented physician-assisted suicide as preferable for two reasons. First, it allows the individual greater personal control over the time and setting of his or her death, something that can have a very beneficial effect. In this regard, he has cited Dr. Quill's patient, Diane, who gained several months of happy and meaningful life because of the reassurance that she could end her life if the suffering and burdens began to dominate her existence. Second, patient control over the decision allows ambivalence to have fuller recognition and expression. The patient can delay if he or she chooses and still have the option of acting on another day. In the Netherlands, if a patient requests that the physician administer the fatal injection and then changes his or her mind, the person runs the risk of being seen as inconsistent in terms of motivation and therefore not an acceptable candidate. Such possibilities clearly can influence the patient to deny his or her ambivalent feelings and comply with the perceived demand characteristics of the situation.

Although proponents of assisted death in the United States seem to prefer assisted suicide as a means to death, there remain those troubling cases of terminally ill individuals who are competent, suffering greatly, and wanting to die, but are too physically compromised or impaired to carry out the act. Thus, for example, a patient with inoperable cancer of the throat and mouth might be unable to swallow the barbiturates prescribed for assisted suicide, or a patient who is almost completely paralyzed might be unable to access the means to end his or her life. Such cases seem to confront us with potentially justified requests for euthanasia. What is our obligation to such patients?

The Arguments Pro and Con

The arguments *pro* and *con* of voluntary euthanasia are, of course, very close to those that are for and against assisted suicide. Proponents base their assertions on the ethical principles of autonomy and mercy. Euthanasia, however, requires the direct involvement of a physician in causing death. The question, then, becomes whether the right to autonomy ever allows or even obligates another person to directly cause death.

As Battin (1994) pointed out, autonomy typically only engenders a patient's right to act freely and without interference. In some circumstances, however, she has argued that a right to self-determination can generate a claim to assistance. Usually, such a claim is acknowledged in cases of handicap or disability. By way of example, our society acknowledges that its citizens have a right to seek an education without interference from others. Yet if someone has a severe physical handicap, such as blindness or deafness, we also recognize an obligation to provide the assistance necessary to allow that person to pursue his or her educational goals. Someone's right to autonomy is not fulfilled if he or she can choose but not act on that choice. So it is if one accepts a so-called right to die. If the patient is terminally ill, is suffering unbearably, has explored all other options for relief, and wants to end his or her life, but is helpless to do so because of physical incapacity, the principles of mercy and autonomy would seem to allow a physician, barring other legitimate moral objections, to aid the patient in bringing about death and an end to suffering in as easy and painless a way as possible.

As with assisted suicide, opponents of euthanasia again argue that the taking of human life is intrinsically wrong, but with euthanasia, they are even more concerned with the so-called slippery slope argument. Their focus is on the potential impact on the physician's adherence to the principles of beneficence and nonmaleficence, as well as on his or her role as healer. In terms of concerns about the so-called slippery slope, it seems obvious that permitting physicians to engage in voluntary active euthanasia could be taking a step toward changing our long-standing moral prohibition against causing the death of another person. Moreover, when another person is responsible for the final act, the possibility of discrimination toward such groups as the elderly, the disabled, or those with a different ethnic background might be more easily introduced. In assisted suicide, it remains the person himself or herself who causes death, but in euthanasia, it is the physician. The fear is that we will not be able to regulate and prevent physicians from engaging in unjustified euthanasia. This fear is, of course, further heightened by the cost containment emphasis in the current health care environment.

For those who believe that life, or at least conscious life, is of value even under the most miserable of circumstances, euthanasia cannot be a benefit, and the physician who performs euthanasia could hardly be seen as acting for the benefit of the patient. In effect, he or she would be seen as violating ethical principles (i.e., beneficence and nonmaleficence) that are central to the role of the physician and would be contributing to the erosion of trust in the physician as healer. Proponents of euthanasia, however, have countered this argument by pointing out that when a suffering person is conscious, whether that experience counts as a benefit overriding his or her suffering is relative to that person and can be decided only by him or her (Battin, 1994).

The Practice of Euthanasia in the Netherlands

Voluntary euthanasia and physician-assisted suicide have been practiced with increased openness in the Netherlands since the 1970s.

Euthanasia has become the preferred form of assisted death and has been supported by public opinion, the majority of physicians, and case law (van der Wal et al., 1996). Despite such support, the Dutch initially devised a system (as mentioned earlier) whereby euthanasia remained a crime punishable by imprisonment, but the medical practitioner was virtually certain that prosecution was avoidable provided that he or she met the appropriate guidelines or *rules of due care*. This system seems to have addressed any concerns that, if it were once officially sanctioned by law, the practice of euthanasia could be subject to serious abuses. The requirements for acceptable practice were formulated by the courts and the Royal Dutch Medical Association, and they were endorsed by a government-appointed commission in 1985. For the mentally competent adult, van der Wal et al. (1996) stated the requirements as follows:

> . . . the patient must consider his or her suffering unbearable and hopeless; the wish to die must be well considered and persistent; the request must be voluntary; the physician must consult at least one other physician; and the physician may not ascribe the death to natural causes and is obliged to keep records. (p. 1706)

From 1990 to 1991, a nationwide study of euthanasia and other medical practices related to the ending of life was commissioned by the Dutch government (van der Maas et al., 1991). At about this same time, the Dutch minister of justice and the Royal Dutch Medical Association agreed on a notification procedure for physician-assisted death that allowed for public oversight of the practice (van der Wal et al., 1996). According to the procedure, a physician who assisted in a patient's death needed to inform the coroner that it was a physician-assisted death and not a natural death. His or her report to the coroner was to be based on an official list of questions about the patient's medical history, the patient's request, the drugs used to cause death, and the report of the other physician who was consulted. The coroner then did a postmortem examination and filed a report of the death and a judgment with the prosecutor general. The case proceeded through successive tiers of the government until the minister of justice made a final decision about whether cause to prosecute or not was present.

In 1995, the government commissioned a second nationwide study to evaluate the practice of euthanasia and to determine whether the notification procedure was serving its purposes of encouraging physicians to disclose cases of assisted death and promoting adherence to the requirements of accepted practice (van der Wal et al., 1996). The investigators who evaluated the practice of euthanasia used two methods, one involving interviews with a sample of 405 physicians and the other involving questionnaires mailed to physicians attending 6,060 deaths that were identified from death certificates. They found that the number of requests for euthanasia had increased since the study in 1990 by approximately 37%, but most of the requests were not granted. With the interview method, 2.3% of all deaths were found to result from euthanasia, as compared to 2.4% with the death-certificate method. In 1990, the rates were 1.9 and 1.7% respectively. The majority of patients involved (approximately 79%) suffered from cancer.

With both the interview method and the death certificate method, it was found that 0.7% of deaths involved ending the patient's life without the patient's explicit concurrent request. In the 1990 study, 0.8% of deaths occurred in this way. Thus, although a slight decline seemed to occur in such cases, it also seems as though even a small number of cases of euthanasia without the request of the patient should be a matter of great concern. This concern is heightened more when it is understood that the actual incidence of such cases is under-reported.

In the study of the notification procedure, van der Wal et al. (1996) estimated that the notification rate had increased from 18% in 1990 to 41% in 1995. Although this increase is substantial, 59% of the assisted deaths were still not reported. Moreover, these investigators found that instances of physician-assisted death without the patient's explicit request were only rarely reported. Of course, the meaning of this finding is that there could have been a far greater incidence than 0.7% of deaths that resulted from euthanasia without the patient's request. These are assisted deaths that have occurred outside of the established legal and regulatory processes. In reported cases of assisted death without patient requests, it was found that in 33% of cases life was shortened by an estimated 24 hours at most, and in another 58% it was shortened by, at most, 1 week. Although this data is meant to be reassuring, we are left not knowing if unreported cases were similarly close to death or what the quality of their lives might have been.

In April 2001, the Dutch Senate voted to legalize euthanasia. The Netherlands thus became the first nation to decriminalize actively ending human life when the requirements for acceptable practice are met. Belgium, a neighbor to the Netherlands, has now followed suit and also legalized the practice (Watson, 2002). The Dutch legislation gives statutory force to voluntary, physician-performed euthanasia, and it allows patients to leave a written request, or advance directive, for euthanasia, should they become too physically and mentally incapacitated to decide for themselves (Weber, 2001). Presumably, the law has resolved the previously uncertain legal situation and has ensured that Dutch physicians acting in good faith and with due care will not face criminal proceedings. Rather than having the public prosecution service decide on whether the accepted criteria have been met, it has empowered regional committees consisting of doctors, lawyers, and ethicists to decide whether a doctor has acted according to the established requirements. It is hoped that making the act legal and placing the immediate review process in the hands of peers rather than prosecutors will enable physicians to feel that they can be more compliant with the reporting process for assisted deaths.

Euthanasia in the United States

Euthanasia is illegal in all 50 states, yet this, of course, does not mean it does not occur. Emanuel, Fairclough, and Emanuel (2000) suggested that it is a relatively rare event. They surveyed nearly 1,000 terminally ill patients at 6 different sites in the United States and estimated that euthanasia and physician-assisted suicide were the causes of death in approximately 0.4% of those who died during the study. In a national survey of physician-assisted suicide and euthanasia that looked at physician practices, however, Meier et al. (1998) characterized euthanasia as not rare in the United States. Likewise, Back et al. (1996), in their survey of physicians in the state of Washington, came to the same conclusion. Among the large sample of physicians in the survey by Meier et al., it was found that the prevalence of having provided a lethal injection was 4.7%. Seven percent of their respondents said that even under current legal constraints, circumstances occur in which they would administer a lethal injection to a competent patient, while 24% said that they would do so if the practice were legal. In every case of actual euthanasia, the physician believed that the request reflected the patient's wishes, and the physicians involved maintained this opinion despite the fact that the final request came from a family member or partner in 54% of the cases. Ninety-six percent of the patients who received a lethal injection were estimated to have less than a week to live, and 59% were considered to be within 24 hours of death.

Orentlicher (1997) argued that the U.S. Supreme Court, by endorsing the practice of terminal sedation in *Washington v. Glucksberg* (1997), has in effect given approval to a form of euthanasia. He has maintained that the withholding of food and water (something that by necessity occurs with terminal sedation) does nothing to relieve the patient's suffering. It only serves to bring about death. From this perspective, it is the state of diminished consciousness, brought on by physician-performed sedation, that renders the patient unable to eat and drink, which in turn results in death.

With the extreme cases in which terminal sedation is considered, we enter (as noted in chapter 3) a morally complex and ambiguous arena (Quill & Byock, 2000). Those who hold that terminal sedation is another example of the double-effect principle have also acknowledged that it strains the boundaries of this principle. Because it poses many of the same risks of abuse as assisted suicide and euthanasia, it would seem equally problematic from an ethical standpoint. Yet it is precisely terminal sedation that the American Medical Association offered, and the U.S. Supreme Court accepted, as an alternative rendering assisted suicide unnecessary in the case of *Glucksberg* (Brief of the American Medical Association et al., 1997).

CONCLUSION

It seems that, for certain cases, a compelling argument for rational suicide can be made. These cases typically have to do with patients who are competent, terminally ill, and suffering greatly without the possibility of relief. Likewise, individual cases exist where strong arguments can be made for assisted suicide or for active voluntary euthanasia. There seem to be grave risks of abuse, however, in legalizing these practices. This statement seems particularly true for euthanasia because it can be performed without the patient's consent, while assisted suicide cannot. In the Netherlands, for example, it is clear that euthanasia without the patient's explicit request has occurred, but it is not clear to what extent and under what conditions it has occurred.

Given the high cost of medical care in the United States and the lack of universal insurance coverage, it seems very reasonable at this juncture to maintain the distinction suggested by Beauchamp and Childress (2001) between a justifiable act and a legitimized practice. In other words, assisted death may be morally justified in certain individual cases characterized by extreme and unrelenting suffering, but until it is clear that abuses can be tightly controlled, it seems best not to press for wider legal sanction. The experiences and developing practices in Oregon and the impact of the legalization of assisted death in the Netherlands provide opportunities to study these issues in greater depth and over a longer period of time prior to reaching any type of closure. It will be of particular interest to see if the legalization in the Netherlands leads to improved reporting practices, if the Dutch can gather better information on the extent to which euthanasia without the patient's consent occurs, and if they can improve efforts to prevent such events from occurring outside of the legal process.

5

THE WISH TO PROLONG LIFE

Well, what is this that I can't see
With ice cold hands takin' hold of me
Well, I am death, none can excel
I'll open the door to heaven or hell
Whoa, death someone would pray
Could you wait to call me another day?

—From the folk song, "O Death," by Ralph Stanley

The individualistic nature of American society, with its great emphasis on self-determination, has given impetus to the *right to die* movement with its resistance to excessive high-tech involvement in, and medical regulation of, the dying process. As much as this movement may represent a longing for a more humanistic approach to the end of life, and the hope for death with dignity, other countervailing forces are present in our society. For some segments of the population, life is felt to have an intrinsic value regardless of any adverse conditions, and hastening death is never desirable. Others hold religious beliefs that ascribe value to whatever suffering one must endure, or they assert that the time of death is not something for men to determine. In addition, our nation maintains the optimistic belief that, through hard work and ingenuity, we can conquer the forces of nature. In the arena of medicine and health care, this belief is manifest in our faith in the power of empirical science and technology, a faith that, as Daniel Callahan (1995) noted, has led us to regard "death as a kind of accident, a contingent event that greater prevention, proven technology, and further research could do away with" (p. 227). As noted in chapter 1, the remarkable advances of biomedical science in the past century have clearly reinforced this perspective.

For those who want to prolong life for as long as possible, the right to die is not a particular consideration. They may encounter conflict, however, when their health care providers believe that life-sustaining treatment is not beneficial and should be withheld or withdrawn. As will be discussed later in this chapter, strong ethical arguments exist on both sides of this conflict. Moreover, many in the medical community expect that a reduction in allegedly futile treatments at the end of life might help to reduce the nation's burgeoning health care expenditures, something for which there is little hard evidence (refer to chapter 1; Emanuel & Emanuel, 1994; Field & Cassel, 1997).

The so-called *futility debate* has been born of this conflict and these expectations. Likewise, there can be a clash of values over the distribution of limited resources for certain highly specialized, life-sustaining treatments and procedures. The *debate over rationing* (i.e., how a treatment is to be allocated when supplies are insufficient for all in need) is the result of this dilemma. In this chapter, we will examine, first, the controversy surrounding so-called futile treatment; second, the issues and problems involved in rationing or the allocation of scarce health care resources; and, third, the related issue of inequities in access to potentially life-prolonging treatments.

THE FUTILITY DEBATE

Some of the issues involved in the futility debate can be illustrated by the classic case of Helga Wanglie (Miles, 1991). Mrs. Wanglie was an 85-year-old, married woman who was taken from a nursing home and hospitalized at the Hennepin County Medical Center in Minneapolis on January 1, 1990. At the medical center, Mrs. Wanglie received emergency treatment for dyspnea (labored breathing) that had resulted from chronic bronchiectasis (inflammation or degeneration of the bronchi leading to the lungs). She was intubated and placed on a respirator. Her condition was such that she could not communicate clearly, but she could acknowledge discomfort and she recognized her family when they visited. After several months, the staff determined that they could not safely wean her from the respirator, and she was transferred to a chronic care hospital. A week later, another effort was made to wean her from the respirator and her heart stopped. She was resuscitated and taken to another hospital for intensive care. She did not regain consciousness and the staff felt that it would be appropriate to consider removing life support systems. The family disagreed and had her transferred back to the Hennepin County Medical Center on May 31st. Tests at Hennepin indicated that she was in a persistent vegetative state as a result of severe anoxic encephalopathy (brain damage secondary to insufficient oxygenation of the blood). She was maintained on a respirator with repeated courses of antibiotics, frequent airway suctioning, tube feedings, and biochemical monitoring.

In June and July of 1990, the patient's clinical team was still of the opinion that treatment was not benefitting her, and they again suggested that it be withdrawn. The patient's husband, daughter, and son insisted that it be continued. Their position was that physicians should not play God, that the patient would not be better off dead, that removing life support showed a moral decay in our civilization, and that miracles can happen. The patient's husband told the staff that his wife had never made any statements about her own preferences concerning life-sustaining treatment. The family declined an offer of counseling, including counseling from their own pastor, and asked that the respirator issue not be discussed again.

A new attending physician reviewed the case in October 1990 and again concluded that Mrs. Wanglie's vegetative state was permanent, and that the respirator was not beneficial in that it could not heal her lungs, palliate her suffering, or enable her to experience the benefits of conscious life. It was noted that neither the hospital nor the county had a financial interest in terminating the treatment because the patient's care was fully covered by insurance.

After an ethics consultation, the hospital decided to go to court to request a decision about whether the staff were obliged to continue treatment. They chose to pursue a two-step process in which they would first ask for the appointment of an independent guardian; then, if the guardian agreed that the respirator was not beneficial, they would ask if they were obliged to continue with the respirator. The patient's husband, however, cross-filed and asked to be named his wife's guardian. In July 1991, the trial court appointed the husband as guardian based on the opinion that he was best able to represent his wife's interests. Given this turn of events, the hospital decided to continue with the patient on the respirator because it was uncertain about its legal status if it decided not to do so. Three days later, despite aggressive care, the patient died of septicemia and multisystem organ failure.

This sad and protracted case and others like it (e.g., the case of *Baby K*, an infant born without a major portion of the brain and kept alive on a ventilator [*In re Baby K*, 1994]) demonstrate that disputes about the futility of treatment are often disputes about values and appropriate goals (Beauchamp & Childress, 2001; Truog, Brett, & Frader, 1992). Mrs. Wanglie's family had a religious orientation that viewed life in itself as sacred. Moreover, they believed that a chance of improvement in her condition could not be absolutely ruled out, and they did not wish to relinquish that chance however small. They may also have been reluctant to accept that Mrs. Wanglie's life was ending, and her continued survival, even if only short term, may have meant a great deal to them. The medical staff, on the other hand, seemed to be of the opinion that the chances of recovery were too insignificant to be given serious consideration, that continued treatment had no health-related goal, and that, according to accepted standards of medical practice, treatment was no longer justifiable. Although no financial loss was experienced by the institution, it would also seem that the staff's concern had to do with distributive justice and the use of resources that might be given to others who could derive medical benefit from them.

In cases like the Wanglie case, whose values and goals should take precedence? Can such a case be viewed as *medically futile* with no further obligation to provide treatment despite the wishes of the surrogate? For whom, and in relation to what, is a treatment considered futile? What exactly is meant by the term futility?

Are Efforts to Define Futile Treatment Futile?

Unfortunately, efforts to define futility of treatment have not been particularly successful. Beauchamp and Childress (2001) noted at least four different conceptualizations: (a) treatment that cannot be performed because of the patient's physical condition; (b) treatment that is statistically very unlikely to be efficacious; (c) treatment that will probably produce only an insignificant outcome; and (d) treatment that is very likely to be more burdensome than beneficial. Other bioethicists have suggested additional possible definitions, such as (a) treatment that would only serve to prolong the dying process and bring no relief to the patient's suffering (Gregory, 1995); (b) treatment that cannot reasonably be expected to improve a patient's quality of life (Tan, 1995); and (c) treatment that has proved useless in the last 100 similar cases (Schneiderman, 1993). An exhaustive search would undoubtedly uncover still other attempts at definition.

No consensus has been established on the applicability of any of these definitions, partly because, in most medical situations at the end of life, nothing is absolute. Rather, there are probabilities or likely outcomes that can have different relevance to the different parties involved. Thus, the patient, the surrogate, the health care staff, and the hospital may all have different thresholds for what is considered futile treatment (Truog et al., 1992).

A well-known case in point is that of *Baby Ryan* (Capron, 1995). Ryan Nguyen was born 6 weeks premature, asphyxiated, and with barely a heartbeat. His physicians at Sacred Heart Hospital in Spokane, Washington, diagnosed him as having brain damage, an intestinal blockage, and kidneys that did not remove toxins from his blood. He was sustained on intravenous feedings and dialysis for several weeks. The doctors felt that the outlook was bleak, but they consulted with a children's hospital in Seattle about the possibility of long-term dialysis for Ryan. The program in Seattle, however, refused to accept him for treatment, and stated that it would be immoral to treat this child and prolong his agony with no likely positive outcome.

Ryan's parents refused to accept the recommendation that their son be allowed to die. Because they feared that the hospital had already decided to remove him from dialysis, they sought and obtained an emergency court order that directed the hospital to take whatever immediate steps were necessary, including renal dialysis, to stabilize and maintain his life. The case drew considerable media attention, and physicians at another children's hospital in Portland, Oregon, offered to accept him for treatment. He was transferred to Portland where the doctors performed surgery to clear Ryan's blocked intestines. He recovered from the surgery and was able to switch to nutrition by mouth. In a month and a half, they were ready to send him home. He no longer required dialysis and seemed free of any permanent neurological deficits. A CT scan showed no structural brain problems.

Cases like that of Baby Ryan highlight the possibility of errors in judgment by the medical staff. It should lead us to be cautious about declarations of futility. At times, a different approach to the problem can lead to markedly different results. On the other hand, it is probably best not to be swayed to too great an extent by the extreme case, such as a case that involves a seemingly miraculous cure. In this regard, the definition that Schneiderman (1993) noted earlier (i.e., that a treatment be taken as futile if it has failed in the last 100 similar cases) seems to have some appeal. It sets a high threshold in that it requires a large number of failed attempts at treatment, but it *last 100)* also gives the medical staff the possibility of limiting the use of treatments *cases* that do not seem beneficial. Truog (1995) referred to Schneiderman's proposal as the "'robust definition' of futility" (p. 128) because it is an effort at a direct solution for cases in which a question of futile treatment exists. He has contrasted it with his own *minimalist* approach, an approach that minimizes the role of the concept of futility in actual medical decision making.

Several authors (e.g., Prendergast, 1995; Truog, 1995; and Truog et al., 1992) pointed out the many problems with the *robust* approach. Thus, Schneiderman (1993) did not indicate how similar these cases must be. Is it sufficient to simply look at the last 100 cases, or must one also consider additional factors such as the patient's age, the etiology of his or her illness, and the presence of other concurrent illnesses? What constitutes a failure? Isn't success or failure in end-of-life cases value based? What source or sources of cases might be considered reliable (i.e., should cases be drawn from personal experience, the experiences of colleagues, or published data)? What makes 100 failures a better threshold for futility than 50 or 200? Isn't such a threshold arbitrary? As can be seen, the potential complexities involved in applying such a rule in practice would make it forbidding.

Such problems with rule-based and definition-based approaches to futility have led to the recommendation (supported by the American Medical Association [AMA]) that these efforts should essentially be abandoned in favor of a case-by-case decision-making process (Plows et al., 1999). Moreover, it has been felt that the term *futility* has too often been used as a conceptual weapon to end discussion and to enable physicians to make unilateral decisions that enforce their power and authority (Truog, 1995).

Rather, at such trying times as those near the end of life, the emphasis should be on attempting to ease the burden of grief and improving communication between patients, families, and the health care staff. These are functions which, incidentally, a psychologist on a health care or palliative care team might be ideally suited to fulfill.

A Proposed Process for Decisions About Futile Treatment

MD's wantit both ways!

Ethically, the dispute over futility is between those who strongly support the principle of autonomy with its emphasis on individual choice and self-determination, and those who argue for the integrity of the practice of medicine and distributive justice (Finucane & Harper, 1996; Truog, 2000). When a patient, or a patient's family, has taken a demand for end-of-life treatment to court, the courts have almost unanimously invoked autonomy and given control of the decision to the patient or to his or her surrogate. The result of such legal opinions has been that health care professionals feel that they are disenfranchised and have no moral weight in the decision-making process. Yet demands for medical treatment require the participation of the medical staff and place obligations on them. Should they not have a significant voice in decisions about such treatment?

Prendergast (1995) and Truog (2000) argued that, indeed, doctors and nurses are not simply there to do the bidding of the patient. They are moral participants in treatment decisions and in the actions that they must take to carry them out. It would destroy the integrity of the practice of medicine were it otherwise. Thus, the major goals of medicine are to heal or cure, if possible, and to reduce suffering. If physicians are forced to do otherwise, they run counter to the goals of their profession. Likewise, physicians are required to maintain high professional standards of competence. If they are required to provide ineffective treatments, they cannot maintain such standards. Clearly, physicians can refuse patient requests for harmful treatments and do so on a routine basis. The principle of nonmaleficence demands it.

Patients and families can insist that clinicians provide them with known medical benefits, that is, services that attempt to cure disease, heal or ameliorate injury, or relieve pain and suffering. Some might also say that patients can expect that the preservation of life will be an intrinsic goal of medical care, but this is problematic. Carried to its logical conclusion, it would mean that physicians could not accept Do Not Resuscitate (DNR) status for a patient, that all dying patients would need to be put on ventilators, and that an all-out effort to save the patient, no matter how debilitated, would need to be made in every case. It would return bioethical thought to a time preceding the *Quinlan* and *Cruzan* cases. Thus, although the preservation of life is assuredly a goal of medicine, it is not always sufficient in itself as a goal.

As noted, patients have a right to expect or demand known medical benefits, but when clinicians believe that they have empirically based evidence for maintaining that a particular treatment will have no medical benefit, they are on sound ethical footing in presenting their opinions. They need to remain aware that these opinions are not entirely objective or value free. Hence, the emphasis should be on informing the patient or surrogate, listening to their perspective and values, and engaging in a shared process of decision making. At the least, clinicians should avoid an adversarial stance in which the effort is to determine that the locus of control for decision making lies with the health care staff and not with the patient and his or her family. Rather, as Prendergast (1995) stated, the effort should be "to identify, understand, and weigh competing interests" (p. 842).

Without a doubt, instances will occur when an impasse exists between the medical staff and the patient or patient's surrogate about whether continued life-sustaining treatment is appropriate or not. In such instances, several commentators on this topic (e.g., Halevy & Brody, 1996; Truog, 2000) have recommended that the clinical staff adopt a procedural rather than a definition-based approach to the problem. A procedural approach means that the staff and the institution engage in a fair and open process of attempting to determine the appropriateness or inappropriateness of continued treatment. Zawacki (1995), with his emphasis on genuine ethical dialogue between individuals at the bedside, paved the way for such a process. His has been a call to abandon the polarized debate and control struggle, and have physician and patient attempt to engage in a process of shared understanding and collaborative planning.

Rather than attempting to rely on an illusive definition of futility, a task force formed by the Houston Bioethics Network, a consortium of ethics committees from hospitals in the greater Houston area, has developed a fair process approach to allegedly futile treatment decisions (Halevy & Brody, 1996). The so-called Houston Policy acknowledges that no policy on futility can be value free and entirely objective. It outlines a series of steps for resolving futility dilemmas on a case-by-case basis. The process gives voice to each of the parties in the dispute (i.e., patient, surrogate, and treatment providers) and enables a thorough institutional review of each case. It insists that physicians may not make unilateral decisions of futility.

Under the policy, when a physician is convinced that, from his or her perspective, a life-sustaining treatment is futile, but the patient or surrogate insists that it be provided, the physician must do several things. First, he or she must discuss carefully with the patient or surrogate the nature of the illness or injury, the prognosis, the reasons for considering the treatment futile, and the available options, including palliative care and hospice care. Then he or she must explain that not providing the intervention does not mean abandoning care that promotes comfort, support, and dignity. The physician should further present the options of transferring treatment either to another physician or to another institution and of obtaining a second, independent medical opinion. Finally, the patient or surrogate is to be offered the assistance of institutional resources (e.g., access to patient care representatives, the bioethics committee, nursing, chaplaincy, and social services).

If the patient does not arrange a transfer and an agreement still cannot be reached, the physician must obtain a second medical opinion from a physician who personally examines the patient. The responsible physician must also present the case, along with all pertinent information, to an institutional interdisciplinary body (e.g., a bioethics committee) for review. The patient or surrogate must be notified about this review, informed of its possible outcomes, and encouraged to be present, or have a representative present, to express his or her views. Although arranging a transfer of treatment remains the patient's responsibility, the patient or surrogate is to be informed again of the possibility of such a transfer.

If the institutional review committee agrees that the treatment in question is medically inappropriate, the treatment, under this policy, could be terminated without the agreement of the patient or surrogate, and a plan for comfort care would need to be initiated. If, however, the institutional review does not concur with the physician's opinion of futility, then orders to limit or end the intervention would not to be accepted as valid, unless, of course, the patient or surrogate subsequently agreed to them.

A similar approach to futility decisions has been recommended by the Council of Ethical and Judicial Affairs of the AMA (Plows et al., 1999) and by the National Ethics Committee of the Veterans Health Administration (VHA, 2000). The VHA report specifically addresses the issue of instituting DNR orders when the patient or surrogate objects, but the physician is of the opinion that CPR will primarily inflict suffering with little or no overall medical benefit. Both groups have maintained that such a fair process between parties is used in our judicial system and is consistent with an ethical approach that attempts to balance the competing values of patient autonomy with respect for the integrity of the medical profession. They have cautioned, however, that the legal ramifications of such a course of action (leading to the withholding or withdrawal of life-sustaining treatment) have not, as yet, been tested in court, and their reports clearly constitute recommendations and are not policy statements. Two states, on the other hand, Texas and California, have now passed statutes (California Probate Code, 2000; Texas Health & Safety Code, 1999) that allow physicians to write DNR orders against the wishes of a patient (or surrogate), provided they follow a fair process approach similar to that mentioned earlier.

In summary, those currently engaged in attempting to resolve so-called futility debates between medical staff and patients (or their surrogates) have moved away from efforts to establish an absolute rule that defines futile treatment. Rather, they are pursuing a *due process* approach that respects the dif-

futility is unsettled

fering opinions of all concerned and requires that the practitioner follow certain procedures in arriving at a decision. Although this approach seems promising and a favorable consensus for it may be building among authoritative groups and agencies, there is as yet no universal agreement that it is an acceptable way to proceed, and, except perhaps in Texas and California, its legal status remains undetermined. Thus, the prudent practitioner in most jurisdictions would be wise to regard this area of practice as still unsettled.

THE DEBATE OVER THE RATIONING OF SCARCE HEALTH CARE RESOURCES

A present risk is that decisions about both futility and the rationing of scarce health care resources can intersect in a negative way. Although, as noted earlier, determinations of futility can be justified on the basis of maintaining the integrity of the practice of medicine, some of the interest in asserting futility has undoubtedly been generated by the need to control health care costs. Likewise, the need to ration scarce and expensive life-sustaining treatments could motivate declarations of futility as a way of limiting the use such resources. It is obviously important to avoid the moral pitfall of using decisions of futility as a covert form of rationing (Plows et al., 1999).

Rationing is a method of allocating limited resources to those who have a need for those resources. When applied to a scarce supply of certain medical treatments and those individuals who need them, rationing has been referred to as *microallocation*. The term *macroallocation* is said to pertain to such things as how much of our national budget is devoted to health care and how resources are allocated within the health care budget itself (Beauchamp & Childress, 2001). A full discussion of the macroallocation of our health care resources is beyond the scope of this book. It is more appropriately considered under the rubric of organizational or administrative ethics (Maddox, 1998). In this section, we will focus on the issue of rationing or allocating scarce treatments (e.g., heart transplants, liver transplants, and intensive care) to patients who are gravely ill and would otherwise die. At the outset of this discussion, it should be noted that no consensus has been established on how such decisions should be made. In fact, deep, value-based divisions prevent an agreement on the relevant criteria, and, particularly in the United States, a general unwillingness to accept that there may be a scarcity of health resources is also an issue.

The Allocation of Organs as an Example of the Ethical Issues Involved in Rationing

The need to limit the provision of particular life-sustaining treatments to some patients, while excluding others, is exemplified in the field of organ transplantation where true scarcity exists. Such scarcity can also occur with other treatments (e.g., the use of intensive care unit [ICU] beds), but because the ethical issues are essentially the same, we will use the process of allocating organs as our primary example.

As medical technology has advanced, the proportion of appropriate transplant candidates has increased, but there has been a persistent shortage of donated organs. Thus, the United Network of Organ Sharing (2001) reported that over 75,000 men, women, and children are on the national organ transplantation waiting list. The disparity between the number of transplants and the number of people listed has grown from less than 5,000 in 1990 to more than 50,000 in 2001. In the year 2000, 5,794 individuals on the waiting list died because the organ they needed was not donated in time.

Although the sale of transplantable organs is prohibited in the United States, the demand is such that a world-wide black market for organs from living donors has sprung up (Delmonico et al., 2002). In certain cases, payments (that were made in another country) have been said to exceed $200,000. The American Society of Transplant Surgeons recently sponsored a meeting of ethicists, organ procurement organization executives, physicians, and surgeons. Their objective was to see if an ethically acceptable pilot trial could be proposed to offer a financial incentive for a family to consent to the donation of organs from a deceased relative (Arnold et al., 2002). This group unanimously rejected the notion of either direct payment or a tax incentive for cadaver organs, because it would violate the ideal of altruism in organ donation and unacceptably commercialize the value of human life. A majority of the panel, however, supported reimbursement for funeral expenses or a charitable contribution as an ethically acceptable approach to increasing the donation of organs. They suggested a pilot project to investigate if such an approach would be acceptable to the public and successful in increasing donations.

As Schmidt (1998) noted, decisions about the allocation of organs are always life and death decisions; that is, there will always be someone on the waiting list who is passed over this time who will not make it to the next time. When a patient is drawing closer to death and can only be saved by receiving an organ transplant, tension mounts for all concerned. How can decisions about who receives a needed transplant be made in a fair and just way?

Decisions about who gets an organ transplant can be divided into three separate steps (Schmidt, 1998). First, the patient must be referred for evaluation to a transplant program. Second, he or she must be admitted to the waiting list for such a program. Finally, the patient must be selected from the waiting list. Observers have noted that most of the selection actually takes place in the first two stages; that is, the *referral* stage and the *admission to waiting list* stage. Nonetheless, there is little systematic information on why some patients are referred and others are not, or on why some patients are accepted to the waiting list and others are not. Acceptance to the waiting list generally reflects judgments of medical suitability and the prospect of a successful transplant. Patients tend to be excluded if they have complicating medical conditions such as diabetes or an incurable infection. On a behavioral level, patients who are judged as likely to have difficulty with postoperative treatment compliance are often excluded. Thus, if the patient cannot tolerate the strong negative side effects of the antirejection drugs and follow the strict postoperative treatment regimen, there will be an early loss of the transplanted organ. Some have argued that it is irresponsible to grant an organ to someone who will be unreliable during the postoperative period while denying others who are more likely to make better use of it. Others have cautioned that these judgments are fraught with difficulty because no reliable predictors have been found for postoperative behavior. According to Schmidt (1998), most transplant surgeons will admit that they make subjective judgments in this regard, and that they sometimes misjudge a case.

Proposed Criteria for Organ Allocation

For those who have been put on the waiting list, various principles have been proposed for the allocation of organs. They could be allocated according to who is in greatest medical need, who will have the most complete restoration of function, who can pay, who is making the greatest societal contributions, who is selected in a randomized process, and so forth. In Europe, an organ sharing network (the Eurotransplant Foundation) has attempted to distribute organs by matching their human leukocytic or HLA antigens, which are responsible for the rejection of foreign tissue (Schmidt, 1998). If the six most important antigens can be matched (and that is not a frequent event in nonrelated individuals), the organ recipient's immune system is very unlikely to recognize the transplanted tissue as foreign and will tolerate it. The problem with this system, however, is that lower-grade matches (i.e., 2–5 matched antigens) show no significant differences in long-term transplant results. Moreover, today even fully mismatched organs can be transplanted successfully with proper immunosuppresive treatment. It therefore seems unfair to pass over certain individuals because of a poor antigen match.

In the United States, Beauchamp and Childress (2001) have argued that, when decisions must be made about the allocation of scarce, nonreusable medical resources, justice demands that primary attention be given to *medical utility* (i.e., to the patient's medical needs and his or her prospects for successful treatment). In general, the Council on Ethical and Judicial Affairs of the AMA has agreed with this position and has specified five factors that may be taken into account in allocation decisions (Clarke et al., 1995): (a) the likelihood of benefit to the patient, (b) the impact of treatment in improving the quality of the patient's life, (c) the duration of benefit, (d) the urgency of the patient's condition, and, in some instances, (e) the amount of resources required for successful treatment. These factors are intended to maximize the number of lives saved, the number of years of life saved, and the quality of life of those saved.

The actual application of each of the Council's five factors can lead to difficulties. These difficulties do not preclude their use for guidance, but indicate that, as criteria, they must be applied with great caution. In the abstract, the first factor, likelihood of benefit, seems sensible and justifiable because, if those who are most likely to benefit are chosen, it would maximize the number of lives saved. The problem, however, has to do with the fact that predictions of outcome in medicine are very imprecise. The Council therefore has recommended that only *very substantial* differences in the likelihood of benefit be considered relevant. An example they give is that it would be more justifiable to prefer a patient with an 80% chance of graft survival over someone with a 10% chance than it would be to prefer a 60% chance over a 40% chance. Smaller differences in probabilities should not be considered discriminating.

In discussing the second factor, the impact of treatment on improving quality of life, the Council seemed to focus more on improvements in functional status and confused that with an improvement in quality of life. As noted in chapter 1, quality of life is a uniquely personal perception and may or may not vary with changes in discrete areas of functioning. It would seem to be very difficult to know if an improvement in functional status would automatically lead the individual to reassess the overall quality (e.g., the meaning and purpose) of his or her life. One may want to consider the likelihood of an improvement in functional status in allocation decisions, but it should be understood that it is not synonymous with an improvement in quality of life. It is also a question whether the likelihood of an improvement in function deserves a status independent from the first factor, the likelihood of benefit from treatment.

The Council pointed out that the third factor, duration of benefit, can be an appropriate consideration in certain situations. They recommended, however, that for this criterion, patients should be assessed according to their own medical histories and prognoses, not according to aggregate statistics based on membership in a group. It is not always appropriate to give scarce resources to those with the longest expected life span. Such an approach could lead to age-based discrimination. Moreover, it is very difficult to predict life span on the individual level. Yet claims to treatment that will bring only a small increase in duration of life may not be sustainable when they require the use of scarce resources that are in great demand.

The fourth factor, urgency of need, was seen by the Council as most applicable in situations of intermittent rather than persistent scarcity. ICU beds, for example, are scarce only intermittently. Giving priority to more urgent cases is justifiable because less urgent cases are likely to gain access fairly rapidly as beds turn over and the scarcity decreases. When scarcity is persistent, as with heart transplants, however, applying an urgency criterion might result primarily in saving those lives that were of extremely poor quality or had very short duration because these would be the lives that were in the most dire straits. In the meantime, the condition of those patients in less urgent need would be at risk of deteriorating and becoming less able to benefit from treatment.

Finally, instances can occur when the amount of resources needed may be a factor in allocation. Thus, if less of a scarce resource is needed with a given individual, it will conserve the resource and maximize the number of other lives saved. Usually, patients who require less of a resource are very likely to benefit from treatment, and the likelihood of benefit would be the relevant criterion for decision making. Yet occasions arise when the ability to benefit from treatment may be equal, but substantial differences exist in the resources required for different people. Thus, if three transplant candidates were equal in most respects, but one needed a heart transplant, one a liver transplant, and one needed both a heart transplant and a liver transplant, it would be justified to give priority to the patients who needed only the heart transplant and only the liver transplant. One would thereby be likely to save two lives rather than one. The Council cautioned, however, that this criterion should be applied only when it is relatively certain that conserving resources will save more lives.

Unacceptable Criteria for Organ Allocation

The Council has also deemed certain potential criteria ethically unacceptable for the rationing of scarce resources. Although health care in the United States, generally speaking, is allocated according to the ability to pay, such an ability is not an ethically acceptable criterion when it comes to the need for scarce and lifesaving resources. Patients should not be denied such treatment based on their lower socioeconomic status. In addition, a patient's social worth or contribution to society usually should not be a consideration in allocation decisions. The term *usually* is included here because, as pointed out by Beauchamp and Childress (2001), situations can occur in which it is moral to give preference to a few who might save many. For example, one might give a treatment preference to the only sailor on a crowded lifeboat who can maneuver and guide the boat to safety. More generally, however, in a pluralistic society, it is difficult to arrive at an agreement on a definition of social worth or contribution. A social worth criterion can also quickly lead to age-based rationing because some argue that the elderly are no longer making positive contributions to the social good. The Council has been clear in stating that such an approach fails to take into account the variations in productivity within older age groups.

There are some patients whose circumstances make successful treatment a challenge. These patients include those who have substance abuse

problems, those who are poor and homeless, those with transportation problems, those who have antisocial or aggressive personality traits, and so forth.
Such factors should not become criteria for excluding patients from treatment. Rather, decision makers should consider the possibility of whether
rehabilitation or additional support might improve the patient's potential to
benefit from treatment. In a similar vein, invoking moral judgments about a
patient's behavioral contributions to his or her illness should not become a
basis for an allocation decision. Thus, it is not appropriate to give an alco-
holic lower priority for a liver transplant, or a smoker lower priority for a heart
transplant, because such decisions ignore the likelihood that such behaviors
may not be totally under voluntary control. Moreover, as the Council on
Ethical and Judicial Affairs has noted, those who otherwise engage in high-
risk behaviors (e.g., hockey players or mountain climbers) are not denied
treatment for injuries sustained in the context of such voluntary activities.

General Guidelines for Deciding on the Allocation of Organs

No universally accepted process has been established for deciding on
the allocation of organs. The AMA Council on Ethical and Judicial Affairs
(Clarke, 1995) has offered some general guidelines. According to the
Council, all patients seeking transplants should be assessed according to the
five ethically appropriate criteria noted earlier. All of these criteria are seen
as appropriate in certain circumstances. When all the potential recipients in
a cohort have been assessed, organs should be allocated according to the criteria and in a manner that will attempt to maximize the number, length, and
quality of lives saved. If, however, patients are at risk of an extremely poor
outcome (e.g., death), they should be given precedence. Thus, all other
things being equal, a patient who can go from 0% to 50% of full functioning
with a transplant should be given preference over a patient who can go from
25% to 75% of full functioning.

It is clear that the application of these five criteria will not always identify the most appropriate candidates for treatment. With some of the criteria,
only very substantial differences are recognized. When candidates appear to
have equal claims on treatment, it is necessary to have another method for
arriving at a decision that provides each possible candidate with an equal
opportunity of becoming an organ recipient. Here the Council has suggested
either a first-come, first-served method for protecting equality or the development of a weighted formula (based on the five criteria) that would allow
for a greater differentiation of those most deserving of treatment.

It is also clear that physicians of patients who are competing for transplants are not in the best position to make impartial decisions. As advocates
for their own patients, they might be inclined to choose them over others,
and if the choice involved two or more of their own patients, it would make
for a conflict of interest. The United Network for Organ Sharing (UNOS)

has provided a centralized process and formula for allocation, but, while it can provide consistency across hospitals and institutions, it has been criticized for lacking flexibility on an individual case level (Clarke, 1995). A more decentralized decision-making process in which each institution establishes its own method of reaching decisions is likely to lack consistency across facilities, but it will allow a more complete consideration of individual case variables. To date, the field has established no clear direction in terms of whether it is preferable to pursue a more centralized or decentralized decision-making process.

THE ISSUE OF INEQUITIES IN ACCESS TO HEALTH CARE

In the preceding sections of this chapter, we discussed the ethical issues for those who want to prolong life either by pursuing treatment that seems futile or by attempting to gain access to scarce medical resources. As sad as the outcome may be for many of these people, they at least have had the opportunity to press their cause. Such is not the case for many people in the United States. As Field and Cassell (1997) noted, "people may have the theoretical right to make their own medical choices, but many do not have the financial access to minimal care necessary for implementation of those choices" (p. 48). Among these people are undoubtedly some of those who self-select out of organ allocation decisions prior to the so-called *referral* stage. Although the United States spends more resources on health care than any country in the world, no social contract, so to speak, provides a basic level of care for all citizens.

The Problem of the Uninsured

American society has generally allowed the distribution of health care resources to be determined by the ability to pay. According to Beauchamp and Childress (2001), about 60% of the U.S. population pays by utilizing employer-based health insurance coverage. An additional 25% have private health insurance or a publicly supported health insurance program such as Medicare or Medicaid. The rest, some 44 million Americans, lack health insurance of any kind. Some of these uninsured people are employed, but by small businesses that cannot afford insurance benefits for their employees. Still others are considered uninsurable by companies that exclude people with poor health or preexisting conditions that suggest the possibility of expensive future claims.

When serious or terminal illness strike patients who are uninsured or underinsured, the patient and his or her family may be faced with some very difficult choices. Under such circumstances, the wish not to be a burden to the family is often heard. Using data from the five hospital Study to

Understand Prognoses and Preferences for Outcomes and Risks of Treatments (SUPPORT), Covinsky et al. (1996) studied the financial impact of serious illness on the patient's family and on the patient's preferences for care at the end of life. They found that in this large sample of seriously ill people, 27% reported either a loss of most or all of the family savings or a change in family plans because of the cost of the illness. Even more concerning, however, they found that those reporting economic hardship on the family were significantly more likely to prefer comfort care over life-extending care. In this regard, the results were similar for both patient respondents and surrogate respondents.

In another large, multisite study by Emanuel, Fairclough, Slutsman, and Emanuel (2000), it was found that nearly 35% of the terminally ill patients in the study had substantial care needs. Substantial care needs were significantly associated with reports that the cost of the patient's terminal illness was a moderate or great economic hardship for the patient's family, and that they or their families had to sell assets, take out a loan, or obtain an additional job to pay for health care costs near the end of the patient's life. A significantly greater number (14.9%) had seriously thought about or discussed voluntary euthanasia or physician-assisted suicide.

The investigators in both of the previous studies concluded that economic hardship ensuing from an illness may often be serious enough to influence patients' decisions about end-of-life care and hastening death. In effect, more patients might want to prolong life were it not for factors such as the financial burden on the family.

The highly individualistic U.S. approach to health care coverage seems to run counter to the notion that it is in society's interest to protect the health of its citizens and, indeed, that society may have some collective responsibility in this regard. As Beauchamp and Childress (2001) pointed out, threats to health may be viewed as similar to threats presented by crime, fire, and pollution. We use collective actions and resources to combat such threats. Is basic health care not a similar type of essential service that should be available to all citizens?

In addition, it has been argued that, because serious disease, injury, or disability creates significant disadvantages for its victims, justice requires that society use its health care resources to counteract these effects. As noted earlier, when an illness worsens and becomes severe, the costs of care can become overwhelming for many people. The illness, of course, can also diminish, and may eliminate, a person's ability to function and personally work toward offsetting these costs. Under such circumstances, fairness would seem to require some societal assistance with health care needs.

As persuasive as such arguments may be, it has remained problematic to specify how a right to health care might be realized in practice. If such a right were interpreted as meaning that every citizen should have equal access to every available treatment, the health care system would rapidly be exhausted. An alternative might be to attempt to ensure a *decent minimum* or adequate level of basic care for everyone. Beauchamp and Childress (2001) envisioned such a decent minimum approach as consisting of two tiers. The first tier would include universal coverage of basic health needs as well as catastrophic health needs, while the second tier would consist of voluntary private coverage for less essential health needs and desires. Such a system would guarantee equal access to basic health care for all, but allow additional coverage based on ability and willingness to pay.

A major problem encountered with such a system is the problem of delineating what should be included in a decent minimum or adequate level of basic care. The state of Oregon made a pioneering effort to try to define a decent minimum of coverage (Cotton, 1992). In 1989, the Oregon legislature passed a Basic Health Services Act designed to ensure that all citizens with a family income below the federal poverty level would have a decent minimum of health care coverage. The Oregon Health Services Commission was charged with producing a ranked priority list of services that would define basic health care. The Commission issued a preliminary list of 1,600 ranked medical procedures that was, in part, based on cost-effectiveness data. The rankings were widely criticized as unjust and seemingly arbitrary. They were subsequently revised after gathering input from experts and from the community through surveys and town meetings. Yet even after revision, they were criticized because they did not allow for differences among patients in the same diagnosis or treatment category (Field & Cassell, 1997). Thus, some patients who fit a high ranking diagnosis or treatment category had features or problems that made them unlikely to benefit from the treatment, while others were in a lower ranking category and had characteristics that gave them a good chance of benefitting from a usually less effective treatment. In short, the ranking scheme did not accommodate for potential differences in benefits based on differences in patient characteristics.

Still other problems developed when the number of those eligible for the Oregon plan exceeded all expectations. As a result, the Commission had to raise the bar, so to speak, in regard to whom they considered eligible (Firshein, 1996). Moreover, many procedures that were clearly needed (e.g., surgery for an incapacitating hernia) still fell below the cutoff line for minimum coverage. In addition, the plan was heavily criticized for ostensibly placing a lower value on the lives of persons with disabilities than on the lives of those without disabilities.

Other states have subsequently attempted to develop a basic benefits package. Perhaps one of the more successful efforts has been that of Hawaii where no ranking of services has taken place. Rather, the state established a State Health Insurance Program (SHIP) that covered everyone between Medicaid and 300% of the poverty level who did not have insurance (Cotton, 1992). Because Hawaii mandated that all employers provide coverage, everyone without other insurance constituted less than 5% of the population. The state had apparently been absorbing the health costs for this segment of the population previously, but under the plan, those covered had access to prevention and primary care, which reduced overall health costs. Circumstances in Hawaii may have been particularly favorable to such an approach. Most states, however, have continued to struggle with this issue.

The Question of Racial Discrimination in Access to Care

Unfortunately, the problems with access to health care are even more complicated than obtaining health insurance coverage for all, or, as Geiger (1996) pointed out, the provision of health insurance alone does not ensure equity. A number of studies, for example, have indicated that race and income had substantial effects on mortality, use of services, and quality of care among patients who were insured under Medicare (Gornick et al., 1996; Kahn et al., 1994; Navarro, 1990). Gorenick et al. (1996) examined the separate effects of race and income on mortality and the use of services for more than 26 million Medicare beneficiaries. They found that, although both race and income played a part, race was the overriding determinant of the differences. Despite such findings, health policy makers and health care providers have not acted assertively to improve African American and other minority patients' access to medical procedures. This situation has persisted partly because the reasons for these racial differences have not been clear. One speculation has been that patients' preferences might explain racial differences.

Ayanian, Cleary, Weissman, and Epstein (1999) studied whether racial differences in access to kidney transplants were explained by patients' preferences. Theirs was a large study of patients with newly diagnosed end-stage renal disease (ESRD) in four regions of the United States. They selected a stratified random sample of African American women, African American men, Caucasian women, and Caucasian men within each region. Patients were interviewed approximately 10 months after they started dialysis and were asked if they had received a kidney transplant and if they wanted to have a transplant. They were also asked how certain they were about that preference and if they had been referred to a transplant center to be tested for their appropriateness to go on a transplant waiting list. Two primary measures of access to kidney transplantation were used: (a) having been referred for evaluation at a transplant center, and (b) having been placed on a waiting list or received a transplant.

The findings indicated that African American patients were less likely than Caucasian patients to want a kidney transplant. However, among patients who wanted a transplant, African Americans remained significantly less likely than Caucasians to have been referred for evaluation, and significantly less likely to have been placed on a waiting list or to have received a transplant. Even among patients who said they were very certain they wanted a kidney transplant, African Americans were substantially less likely to have been referred, to have been placed on a waiting list, or to have received a transplant. The investigators in this study controlled for coexisting illnesses and various other possible confounding variables, such as health status and perceptions of care, yet the outcome remained essentially unchanged. They concluded that racial differences in access to renal transplantation are pervasive.

The results reported by Ayanian et al. (1999) have been supported by another recent study (Schulman et al., 1999) in which simulated cases with various types of chest pain and similar clinical characteristics were presented. Physicians in this study were found to be less likely to recommend cardiac catheterization for women and African Americans than for men and Caucasians. In addition, there have been studies such as that by Peterson, Wright, Daley, and Thibault (1994) in which the investigators reviewed the discharge abstracts of 33,641 male patients treated for acute myocardial infarction (AMI) in the VHA during the years 1988 to 1990. In the 90 days after admission, they found that African Americans with an AMI were 33% less likely than Caucasians to have undergone cardiac catheterization, 42% less likely to have received coronary angioplasty, and 54% less likely to have received coronary bypass surgery. Among those patients who underwent catheterization, African Americans were also less likely than Caucasians to have had a subsequent revascularization procedure. These results were found after adjusting for patient characteristics such as age, the number of secondary diagnoses, and hospital characteristics, including medical school affiliation and on-site cardiac surgery facilities.

The authors of this study concluded that African Americans in the VHA had lower cardiac procedure use than Caucasians following acute myocardial infarction. The differences in procedure use were not accounted for by differences in disease prevalence, contact with the medical community, or insurance coverage. They speculated that there could have been racial differences in disease severity that were not detected with the use of a secondary database, or that physicians may have believed that African Americans had worse survival rates than Caucasians after such procedures as coronary bypass surgery (a belief, which they pointed out, has not been supported by multiple reviews of surgical outcomes). They also suggested that, within complex physician-patient interactions, a physician's racial and cultural biases could possibly have influenced the decision-making process.

The fact that there have been racial disparities in access to treatment even in a free care system like the VHA, has led some commentators (e.g., Geiger, 1996) to suggest that there may be racially discriminatory rationing by physicians and health care institutions, while others (e.g., Freeman & Payne, 2000) have asserted it more directly. All agree that, if it exists, it has not been conscious or overtly intentional. Nonetheless, the disparity in care is something that is seriously harmful to the health and lives of minority patients.

CONCLUSION

With regard to the wish to prolong life, perhaps Shakespeare, with his great understanding of human nature, said it best in Hamlet's famous soliloquy (*Hamlet*, III, i):

> The undiscover'd country, from whose bourn
> No traveler returns, puzzles the will,
> And makes us rather bear those ills we have
> Than fly to others we know not of?

There is an understandable hesitance about accepting death, and, as mentioned earlier, this hesitance may be reinforced by a number of factors in American culture. As noted throughout this chapter, the major ethical issues involved in decisions to prolong life have to do with autonomy, justice, and the integrity of the medical profession. Although these principles can provide general guidance, they are sometimes difficult to apply in the specific case. Whether it is a decision related to the futility of treatment or to the rationing of scarce resources, it seems most important to remember that we do not as yet have a definitive way to proceed in the decision-making process. Decisions are, in fact, often value based rather than based on any ostensible objective criteria. It is crucial for those involved in these decisions to bear this in mind and, when possible, to engage in a meaningful dialogue and effort to resolve any emerging conflicts with patients. Engaging in a control or power struggle with terminally ill patients or their families typically leads to difficult and bitter feelings. On the other hand, much can be gained by pursuing a fair process in which the views of all parties are respected.

On a larger level, it is also important that we remain cognizant of the fact that many in the United States do not have equal access to life-prolonging medical services because they are uninsured, poor, or belong to a less privileged or minority group. As noted in chapter 1, African Americans, on average, live 6 years less than Caucasian Americans (Centers for Disease Control, 1999). In this regard, Geiger (1996) called for "the routine and ongoing examination of racial disparities in the use of services and in choices of diagnostic and therapeutic alternatives" (p. 816) through the quality assurance protocols of every hospital. He also suggested that the dilemma of race and health care be made a part of every physician's training.

Access to the care that an individual would want near the end of life goes hand in glove with the settings and health care programs that have been developed. In this regard, it is a sensitive community that attempts to create choices for its citizens (Maddox, 1998). Our next chapter is a discussion of the alternative settings and systems of care that are available in the United States for patients near the end of life.

6

ALTERNATIVES IN CARE
NEAR THE END OF LIFE

Some people are lucky and go, zip—heart attack or brain hemorrhage and they're gone. That's lucky. I've worked in hospitals enough that I know what it's like to lay there. I worked as a nurse's aide for five years at Mercy Hospital in Jackson, Michigan. I remember taking care of cancer patients who smelled so bad when you'd go in the room that you'd just have to paste a look on your face to keep them from knowing.

—Peggy Terry in S. Terkel (2001), pp. 255–256

Jay chose to die at home, and I would pray for him to die because of the pain he was in. He was thirty-six years old, my age today. He was losing his mind. He was a brilliant person. . . . He didn't want to go to the hospital. His care was at home. . . . I learned how to give him injections, I learned how to change his IVs, and I learned how to just try to cope with it day to day.

—Tico Valle in S. Terkel (2001), p. 276

    Not only has the prospect of modern dying, with its prolonged and, at times, technology-driven trajectory, given rise to concerns about the manner and time of death, it has also given rise to concerns about end-of-life care. Profoundly disturbed by the apparent insensitivity to the needs of dying patients by her acute care-oriented and cure-driven medical colleagues, a British physician, Cicely Saunders, initiated modern hospice care in England in the 1960s (Butterfield-Picard & Magno, 1982). *Hospice* is a term that was originally used in the Middle Ages to refer to a place of shelter for sick and weary travelers returning from religious pilgrimages. Dr. Saunders adopted this term for the place, St. Christopher's Hospice, near London, where she provided comfort care for dying patients. Drawing on Dr. Saunders' work, the first hospice program in the United States was begun in New Haven, Connecticut, in 1974. Since then, the growth of the hospice movement has been remarkable. By 1981, over 800 hospice programs were active in this country (VandenBos, DeLeon, & Pallack, 1982), and today reportedly over 3,000 are in existence (Hospice Foundation of America, 2002, February 20).

The emergence of the hospice movement has been a direct response to perceived inadequacies in care for dying patients. For much of human history, dying was generally a family and community event, not a medical one. Currently, in the United States, however, death at home and in the care of the family has been replaced, in large measure, by death in a more impersonal institutional setting. As the Institute of Medicine's Committee on Care at the End of Life has stated, "Death is not what it used to be" (Field & Cassel, 1997, p. 33). Thus, in 1949, it was estimated that nearly 50% of deaths occurred in institutions, primarily hospitals and nursing homes. By 1958, the estimate had risen to 60.9%, and by 1980 it was said to be 74%. In 1992, the estimate remained at 74%, but the number of deaths in nursing homes increased modestly, and the number of deaths in hospitals declined modestly.[1] This leveling off and shift in distribution has been attributed to the fact that Medicare began to cover hospice services in 1983, and at the same time Medicare also began to encourage the reduced use of inpatient hospitalization (Field & Cassel, 1997).

The setting in which one dies can have a significant influence on the care that one receives. The setting and the services provided, however, can be markedly changed by the system of care that is employed in any particular setting. In this chapter, we discuss the systems of care and the settings (primarily hospitals, nursing homes, and at home) in which Americans die. We also discuss recent efforts to extend hospice-like changes in our medical system of care to those who have an advanced illness, that is, those at a stage in the disease process that precedes terminal illness.

CONVENTIONAL CARE AND HOSPICE CARE

The Conventional Approach

Conventional care (CC) for dying patients does not refer to a system of care that specifically focuses on the needs of terminally ill patients. It refers to dying within the traditional medical care system in the United States. The traditional system, for the most part, has been acute care oriented and cure

---

[1] It is noteworthy that significant state-by-state variations exist for in-hospital death rates. The state of Oregon, for example, has reported that less than one third of the deaths in that state occur in hospitals, while it has the highest rate of any of the other states for deaths at home (Wyden, 2000).

driven. It tends to view death as a failure. When medical and technological efforts are unable to alter a patient's terminal course, a tendency to avoid that individual becomes prevalent, except for the delivery of essential services. The system rewards those practitioners who wish to bring about advances in combating illness and in utilizing the latest technology. As a result, very little support exists for treatment and research in the palliative care area of practice (Lattanzi-Licht & Connor, 1995).

There can be little doubt, however, that within our CC system large numbers of dying patients and those with advanced illnesses suffer from unrelieved pain and other symptoms, such as difficulty in breathing, vomiting, sleeplessness, and mental confusion. In reviewing evidence for unrelieved symptoms in dying patients, the Committee on Care at the End of Life found that moderate to severe pain had been reported in 30 to 50% of patients with advanced cancer, HIV/AIDS, and multiple sclerosis (Field & Cassel, 1997). In the large, prospective SUPPORT study that examined a range of diagnoses (nine in all) in seriously ill hospitalized patients, it was reported that 90% of patients with chronic obstructive pulmonary disease and 70% of patients with lung cancer or multiple organ system failure suffered from severe dyspnea (very labored breathing) in the three days prior to death. In this same study, 25 to 30% of patients with cirrhosis, colon cancer, and lung cancer were found to suffer with severe confusion (Lynn et al., 1997).

Findings such as these have led Lynn and her colleagues (e.g., Introcaso & Lynn, 2002; Lynn et al., 2002) to express the need for multisite collaboration in the use of quality improvement methods as a way of reforming end-of-life care in conventional settings. These authors have recommended repeated quality improvement cycles across institutions in which a problem is identified (e.g., slow response time to complaints of shortness of breath), a plan for improvement is generated, success is measured, and, based on the results, further action is developed.

Although certain strategies are effective at symptom relief, the Committee on Care at the End of Life found substantial evidence in the research literature of the undertreatment of pain and other symptoms (Field & Cassel, 1997). In part, pain management and the management of dyspnea in a conventional setting may be compromised by widespread physician concerns about prescription drug laws that are meant to discourage drug addiction and the diversion of drugs from legal to illegal sources. Thus, for example, regulatory policies and laws often put limits on the number of dosages of a controlled substance that may be prescribed at any one time. This forces the severely ill and dying patient to inconvenience his or her physician and request frequent renewals of prescriptions. For terminal patients who have inconsistent assistance at home, this can lead to interruptions in pain and symptom management.

As if physician concerns about prescription drug laws were not enough, Werth (2002) predicted that U.S. Attorney General John Ashcroft's recent

efforts to oppose the Oregon Death with Dignity Act (ODDA) by reinterpreting the Controlled Substances Act, if successful, will lead physicians to
be even less likely to provide adequate types and doses of pain medication to
terminally ill patients. In effect, his proposal would criminalize actions
related to the provision of controlled substances (e.g., opioids) if a patient
dies and external observers believe that the physician's intent was to hasten
the patient's death. Werth hypothesized that many physicians will avoid
doing anything that might lead to their intent being questioned; hence, it is
likely that prescriptions would decrease for controlled substances in situations
where death is near.

No known evidence proves that the prescription of opioids for pain control in dying patients leads to any significant drug diversion problems.
Moreover, the use of opioids for pain may produce drug tolerance and physical dependence in terminal patients, but this should not be equated with
addiction or drug abuse, something that is more associated with continued and
compulsive use despite harmful effects (Gilson & Joranson, 2002). In this
regard, the Committee on Care at the End of Life and others such as the Pain
and Policy Studies Group at the University of Wisconsin–Madison (Joranson,
Gilson, Dahl, & Haddox, 2002) have recommended that states pass carefully
crafted laws that define addiction. They also suggest that states provide physicians and patients with the protection needed to feel comfortable in treating
intractable pain occurring within the context of a terminal illness.

Access to adequate pain medication may be an even greater problem for
minority groups who receive care at home. Thus, Morrison, Wallenstein,
Natale, Senzel, and Huang (2000) surveyed a randomly selected sample of
30% of New York City's pharmacies. After an analysis that adjusted for age
and rates of burglary, robbery, and drug-related arrests, they found that pharmacies in predominantly non-Caucasian neighborhoods were significantly
less likely to stock opioids than pharmacies in predominantly Caucasian
neighborhoods. The investigators concluded that non-Caucasian patients
may be at great risk for undertreatment of pain. They called for programs to
educate pharmacists about safe and appropriate ways to use and supply opioid analgesics.

Given that the undertreatment of pain is a serious problem in the
United States, routine screenings and assessments are needed in hospitals,
nursing homes, and during home care (HC). Certainly among those with
advanced or terminal illness, pain should be treated aggressively.[2] In terms of

[2]The undertreatment of pain and other symptoms is a serious problem in end-of-life care, but for those
who are severely ill, difficulties can also occur in attaining an acceptable balance between the control of
pain and the maintenance of mental alertness and clarity. Under some circumstances, the dosages of sedatives and analgesics needed to relieve pain may cause the patient to be so drowsy that he or she is unable
to be as aware of the presence of loved ones as he or she would like. Those who monitor pain must also
be sensitive to the patient's and family's wishes in terms of sedation and must attempt to titrate dosages
to achieve the most tolerable levels of pain control and mental acuity.

screening for pain, a program called *Pain: The 5th Vital Sign* has been an encouraging development in the Veterans Health Administration (VHA) (Department of Veterans Affairs, 2000). This program has attempted to train doctors and nurses to treat screening for pain like a vital sign, that is, like something that is routinely checked as part of good clinical practice. Thus, a positive pain score on a numeric rating scale (0 being no pain and 10 being the worst possible pain) prompts for further assessment and possible intervention.

Hospice and Palliative Care

It has been a reaction to the difficulties noted earlier in the CC system that has given rise to the hospice system. At times, the term hospice has been taken to refer to a place of care, or to a system or philosophy of care for dying patients, or even to a social movement about changing the nature of medical care itself. Although Cecily Saunders' early hospice work was associated with a place in which patients received care (St. Christopher's Hospice), most hospices today deliver care in a variety of settings and emphasize in-home care. There seems little doubt that Dr. Saunders intended to create a comprehensive model of terminal care that transcended the setting in which care was given.

As it has developed, the conceptual framework for hospice care has come to differ from the traditional models of care for terminally ill patients in a number of significant ways (Butterfield-Picard & Magno, 1982). First, to the greatest extent possible, hospice care attempts to place decision making in the hands of the patient and his or her family. This emphasis is in contrast to the traditional medical model in which the physician is the primary decision maker. Second, acute care or cure-directed interventions (such as chemotherapy or radiation treatment) are generally considered inappropriate because they cannot stop the advance of truly terminal illness, and they often cause great physical and mental suffering with an associated loss of dignity. Third, palliative care is the major focus of the hospice approach. Palliative care seeks to relieve, reduce, soothe, or prevent the symptoms of disease or disorder without bringing about a cure. It stresses the control of pain and the relief of suffering. Fourth, hospice care is provided by an integrated, multidisciplinary team that includes physicians, nurses, psychologists, social workers, spiritual counselors, health aides, and volunteers. Fifth, the hospice program endeavors to diminish any sense of the emotionally sterile, clinical environment of an institution while encouraging the maintenance of normal, home-like surroundings. Finally, family members are offered bereavement counseling after their loved one has died.

The hospice approach encourages people to confront the dying process openly and as the inevitable and natural final phase in the life cycle. It provides support and care so that a dying person can live as fully as possible until death occurs. It does not attempt to shorten life; however, it strives for a death that is as comfortable as possible and free of needless and futile technological efforts to prolong life. It values personal autonomy in decision making and tends to view the more traditional, paternalistic medical model of care as inappropriate for the needs of dying people.

In the early 1980s, great interest in the United States was devoted to the possibility of introducing this type of care for dying patients as an option for Medicare reimbursement. Although hospices were developed to improve care rather than reduce costs, some of their appeal in political circles was that they seemed to provide more appropriate care and be less costly. At this same time, a group at Brown University undertook what came to be known as the National Hospice Study (Greer & Mor, 1986). The study was designed to compare the costs and benefits of hospice care with nonhospice terminal care. A total of 1,754 terminal cancer patients and their primary care persons (PCPs) from 14 CC settings and 40 hospices took part in the study. The hospices included both those without inpatient beds (HC) and those with inpatient beds (hospital-based care, HB). The patients and their PCPs were interviewed regarding the patient's condition, quality of life, symptoms experienced (particularly pain), and services provided. The interviews took place at study entry, 7 days after study entry, and every 2 weeks thereafter. The investigators used several standardized measures of functional performance, quality of life, and severity of pain. Because the proportion of patients able to respond to questions dropped as death approached, the interviews with the PCPs were viewed as providing continuity of measurement over the course of the study (Greer et al., 1986).

The pertinent findings in this large prospective study were that hospice patients received fewer aggressive forms of treatment (such as chemotherapy, surgery, or radiation therapy) and fewer diagnostic tests. They also received more care at home and spent fewer days in the hospital in their last month of life. The total cost per day was substantially lower in HC hospices, but the costs of HB hospices were equivalent to the costs of CC. Pain and symptom control were found to be better in HB hospices as opposed to CC sites. Patients in HB hospices were more likely to have analgesics prescribed and to actually receive them on a regular schedule. Thus, it seemed that HB hospices closely monitored pain and calibrated treatment accordingly (Morris et al., 1986). The HB hospice PCPs reported higher satisfaction with the patient's care than conventional care PCPs, and PCPs in both types of hospices were more satisfied with where the patients died. Surprisingly, however, no significant differences were found between hospice and CC systems on quality of life measures.

The null findings on quality of life led some to question whether a reevaluation of the claims made for hospice care was needed, whereas others questioned whether the traditional measures of quality of life really captured the impact of hospice care. Wallston, Burger, Smith, and Baugher (1988) took the latter approach. Their thinking was that hospice care strives to give people the opportunity to die as they choose and to gain some control over where, under what circumstances, and with whom they will die. Based on this thinking, they devised a quality of death measure that was applied to a subset of patients from the National Hospice Study who had PCPs who participated in a bereavement interview between 90 and 120 days after the patient's death.

The quality of death measure consisted of 13 situational elements that were derived from the interviews of all patients in the National Hospice Study when they were admitted to the study. These patients were asked what they would like their last 3 days of life to be like. The derived elements were weighted according to the number of patients who mentioned a given element. Among the elements were items such as (a) the people whom he or she wanted were there, (b) physically able to do what he or she wanted, (c) freedom from pain, (d) feeling at peace or happy, and so forth. The PCPs were asked to determine whether each of these 13 elements were present or absent during the final 3 days of the patient's life. The results indicated that the quality of death scores were significantly lower for those receiving CC as compared to those in either type of hospice care (HC or HB). Differences between the two types of hospice care were not significant. Although their study has limitations, the investigators concluded that their results supported the impression that hospice care optimizes the quality of death for terminally ill patients.

The National Hospice Study was intended to provide data for health policy planners to use when deciding on third-party funding options (Greer & Mor, 1985). Before the study was completed, however, Congress had already passed legislation, the Tax Equity and Fiscal Responsibility Act (1982), making hospice a federal program reimbursable under Medicare. The availability of Medicare and Medicaid benefits to hospice patients became the engine that drove the growth of the hospice movement in the United States. Thus, although there are still many small, volunteer, HC hospices, many hospice programs have developed into professional organizations for large numbers of dying patients in a variety of settings (Lattanzi-Licht & Connor, 1995).

In spite of the tremendous growth of the hospice movement, it has remained, in many ways, outside the mainstream of the health care system. The initial hope of those involved was that hospice values and palliative care would become routine in terms of medical care for dying patients. In fact, some efforts have been made to develop palliative care programs within the hospital setting. These programs have been designed for patients who are not only terminally ill but also for those who are severely ill but not yet terminal (Haley, Niemeyer, Larson, Kwilosz, & Kasl-Godley, 2003). Despite the promise of such programs and units, the leaders of the medical profession have not embraced them. As Lattanzi-Licht and Connor (1995) pointed out, work done in hospice and palliative care programs in the U.S. medical system tends to be viewed as something undertaken by those who lack the drive and ability to explore the frontiers of medicine. Moreover, efforts to have palliative medicine recognized as a medical specialty have met with great resistance.

Such, however, has not been the case in Great Britain, where hospice programs have been more widely embraced by the medical establishment. Palliative medicine is now recognized as a specialty, and career posts have been established. A number of well-regarded physicians are conducting credible research on symptom management. They are accumulating what is becoming an impressive body of knowledge on palliative medicine. It would seem that something similar will need to happen in the United States if hospice and palliative care are to become better integrated into the health care system. Of course, this is not to deny that many inroads have been made. Hospice care can now be offered in all the major settings in which Americans die.

THE HOSPITAL SETTING

In the United States, more deaths occur in hospitals than in any other setting, yet hospitals, in general, have been organized to cure illnesses, save lives, and maintain control over death (Benoliel & Degner, 1995). Thus, there is an apparent conflict between the traditional hospital setting and the dying patient; that is, as noted earlier, death represents failure to the cure ethic of most hospitals. It has become a major challenge to hospitals to maintain their efforts at fighting illness and prolonging life while also attempting to avoid such heroic actions with those patients who are beyond saving and primarily need comfort care. Typically, the services needed to meet the needs of dying patients and their families are seen as secondary to the life-saving activities of the hospital.

The shortcomings in hospital care for dying patients have been clearly documented in studies such as the large, prospective Study to Understand Prognoses and Preferences for Outcomes and Risks of Treatment (SUP-PORT) (The SUPPORT Principal Investigators, 1995). This study was designed, first, to observe and understand HB care for patients with advanced illnesses and, second, to identify opportunities for improvements in care. In the observational phase, the investigators noted that the final hospitalization for half the patients in their sample included more than 8 days in generally undesirable circumstances or conditions, such as being in an intensive care unit (ICU), receiving mechanical ventilation, or being comatose. According to the families of patients who were able to communicate, nearly half of them spent half their time in moderate to severe pain during their final days. Discussions and decisions in advance of death were infrequent. Only half the physicians knew when their patients preferred to avoid cardiopulmonary resuscitation (CPR), and nearly half of all Do Not Resuscitate (DNR) orders were not written until the last 2 days of life.

This apparent neglect of those who die in hospitals has led the Committee on Care at the End of Life to raise a number of basic issues and questions to be considered by hospitals concerned with improving the care of terminally ill patients (Field & Cassel, 1997). The Committee essentially asked hospitals to examine their own performance in regard to the degree to which they carry out activities such as the following:

- Inform patients and families about who is responsible for their care, what they can expect, and to whom they can look for information and assistance
- Focus on advance care planning and determine the preferences of patients and families
- Make internal and external expertise available to clinicians, patients, and families relative to symptom evaluation and management, decisions about withholding or withdrawing treatments, bereavement support, and so forth
- Train hospital personnel in methods of communicating bad news and respecting dignity
- Train ICU staff and other personnel to recognize patients for whom goals of curative or life-prolonging care should be reconsidered
- Follow guidelines, symptom assessment protocols, and other tools that guide clinical evaluation and care for different kinds of patients who are likely to die
- Make care options such as a designated area of palliative care beds available to dying patients
- Assist patients and families with transitions to or from the hospital and other care settings such as nursing homes, HC agencies, and hospices
- Reliably document and update advance planning decisions, symptom assessments, care processes, and so forth
- Prevent or mediate conflicts among clinicians, patients, families, and others through structures like an ethics advisory committee (EAC)
- Evaluate and improve the quality of care given to dying patients

Although the Committee acknowledged that there is wide variability among hospitals in terms of the constraints that they face in attempting to improve care for dying patients, it nonetheless noted that "the message of this report is that each hospital should be held accountable for identifying its shortcomings and devising strategies to improve the quality and consistency of care at the end of life" (Field & Cassel, 1997, p. 99).

Perhaps the message to terminally ill patients and their families and advocates is to inquire about the extent to which their hospital of choice has endeavored to meet the recommendations of the Committee. Moreover, if it is clear that HB care will be needed in the course of dying, the patient and his or her family may wish to explore the possibilities of associating with a hospital-based hospice program in which it can be assured that palliative care principles will be brought to the hospital setting.

THE NURSING HOME SETTING

As noted at the beginning of this chapter, a modest increase in the number of deaths in nursing homes and a modest decrease in the number of deaths in hospitals have been observed in recent years. According to Zerzan, Stearns, and Hanson (2000), the probability that a nursing home would be the site of death increased from 18.7% in 1986 to 20.0% in 1993. It is expected that this trend may only increase in future years as the number of older people grows and as efforts to minimize hospital stays continues. Given the nature of the elderly and functionally impaired population found in nursing homes, one might think that nursing homes would be well prepared to care for dying patients. Such is often not the case, however. In fact, the Committee on Care at the End of Life found that nursing homes and other long-term care organizations were deeply challenged by end-of-life care and decision making (Field & Cassel, 1997).

The difficulties that nursing homes have with end-of-life care may be attributable to several factors. First, federal policy has emphasized rehabilitation and the restoration of function, or reaching the highest level of functioning possible, as the goals of nursing home care (Blevins & Deason-Howell, 2002). Medicare, for example, provides higher reimbursement for restorative care and less reimbursement for the intensive personal care and symptom management needed for terminally ill patients (Zerzan et al., 2000). Thus, palliative care functions like pain and symptom management tend to be underemphasized. Moreover, nursing homes are more likely to view some of the natural processes of dying (such as the loss of appetite and weight loss) as medical problems to be overcome. Second, the staff in nursing homes is usually not trained in providing palliative care. There is a relatively low level of physician involvement as well as a relatively low ratio of registered nurses to residents or patients. Much of the day-to-day care is provided by licensed practical nurses and nursing assistants or aides who tend to be less well trained and poorly paid for very hard work (Benoliel & Degner, 1995; Field & Cassel, 1997). Finally, because nursing homes must provide the very basic services of bathing, feeding, dressing, and mobilizing a large number of frail, confused, and disabled people, the work tends to become regimented. Often little time is available for the personalized care needed by dying patients.

The Committee on Care at the End of Life has stated that "it is essential to direct more explicit and open attention to the manner of dying in nursing homes and the ways in which care can be improved for dying patients"

(Field & Cassel, 1997, p. 100). Evidence based on the perceptions of family members shows that hospice care in nursing homes improved both physical and emotional symptom management and reduced the need for hospitalization (Baer & Hanson, 2000). Yet nursing home residents who are dying have only limited access to palliative and hospice care. Despite the fact that the Medicare hospice benefit includes residents of long-term care facilities, 70% of nursing homes have no hospice patients (Zerzan et al., 2000).

Part of the problem seems to have financial roots. Patients covered under Medicare alone may select a conventional skilled nursing benefit following an acute hospital stay or a hospice benefit, if they are terminally ill. The choice, however, is not financially neutral. The Medicare skilled nursing benefit covers room and board, while, under the hospice benefit the resident must pay room and board. Thus, the financial incentive is clearly not in favor of hospice care (Zerzan et al., 2000). Nursing home residents who actually receive hospice care are typically those who have become eligible for both Medicare and Medicaid. Once a resident's savings have been spent down to the poverty level, he or she becomes eligible for Medicaid, which covers the costs of room and board at a rate of 95% of the regular daily expense (Blevins & Deason-Howell, 2002). The choice between hospice care and skilled nursing care is then possible without substantial negative financial consequences.

A second part of the problem has to do with the fact that for a resident to qualify for the Medicare hospice benefit, a physician must certify that the resident has 6 months or less to live. As noted in chapter 3 of this volume, however, Christakis and Lamont (2000) found that 63% of doctors, when asked for prognoses upon referring patients to a hospice, were overly optimistic in their predictions for survival, while only 20% of the physicians were considered accurate (with accuracy defined as between .67 and 1.33 times the actual length of survival). Undue optimism about survival prospects is a likely contributor to late referrals for hospice care. Moreover, physicians' ability to predict the time until death is perhaps best when a primary diagnosis of cancer has been made. It is far less certain with other diseases, and physicians are less likely to want to offer predictions. Nursing home residents tend to die of heart disease and stroke more frequently than cancer. The 6-month prognosis requirement is therefore a challenge with many nursing home residents, and access to hospice care is consequently more limited, even though many residents might prefer a palliative approach to care.

Finally, under Medicare regulations, the hospice program assumes overall responsibility for the management and implementation of the care plan for the terminal illness. The nursing home staff must continue to provide their usual services to the patient, but must relinquish control over many aspects of care. Under such circumstances, nursing homes are likely to view hospice staff as interfering with their work, or as yet another level of unwanted oversight, and choose not to offer access to a hospice program (Zerzan et al., 2000).

Both the Committee on End of Life Care (Field & Cassel, 1997) and Zerzan et al. (2000) made recommendations for improving care for patients dying in nursing homes. These recommendations have included increased education and training in palliative care, as well as heightened emphasis on pain and symptom assessment and management, for all nursing home staff. It has also been recommended that financially neutral reimbursement mechanisms be developed for nursing home hospices under Medicare. Moreover, it has been suggested that demonstration projects be initiated to test the cost-effectiveness of hospices as palliative care consultation services in nursing homes. Hospice care could then be made available through consultation to those who do not necessarily meet the 6-month prognostic criterion.

THE HOME SETTING

Dying at home has all the possible advantages of being in close communication with loved ones and being in familiar surroundings during one's final days. It comes as no great surprise, however, that terminally ill patients who remain at home have wide-ranging needs for assistance in addition to the medical care that they receive from physicians. In a national sample of terminally ill patients recruited through physicians' offices, Emanuel et al. (1999) found that 86.8% of their sample needed some assistance, and 34.7% required substantial assistance with transportation, nursing care, homemaking, and personal care. Half the patients in this study (50.2%) reported that they were experiencing a moderate or greater amount of pain, 17.5% were bedridden more than half the day, 70.9% reported shortness of breath when walking one block or less, 35.5% had urinary or fecal incontinence, and 16.8% reported symptoms of depression.

It also undoubtedly comes as no surprise that nearly three quarters (72.1%) of the primary care givers for this population were women, that is, for the most part, wives or partners, daughters, and sisters. In our society, it is still women who are predominantly called on to provide care for dying people. For unskilled assistance with transportation and homemaking, most patients relied on family and friends (76.8% for transportation and 66.3% for homemaking). Even for care of a skilled nature (such as nursing care), a large number looked to family and friends for assistance. Thus, in terms of nursing care, 42.4% received care only from family and friends, while 28.3% used a combination of family, friends, and paid assistance. Approximately 24.2% used only paid assistance.

Home Care and Hospice Care

For patients in the study by Emanuel et al. (1999) who used paid help, the vast majority were enrolled in a hospice program or a home health care agency. Hospices in the United States were, of course, originally intended to help people die at home rather than in the unfamiliar and sterile surroundings of an institution. Hospices generally make a commitment to be accessible to dying patients and their families 24 hours a day and 7 days a week. Most home hospices emphasize the need for a family member or a close friend who is willing to serve as a primary caregiver. Some will not accept patients without someone who can fulfill this key role in the team effort.

The caregiver role, however, can be very demanding and stressful. Haley, LaMonde, Han, Narramore, and Schonwetter (2001) found that spousal caregivers of hospice patients who had either dementia or lung cancer had higher rates of depression, lower life satisfaction, and poorer physical health than age-matched, noncaregiving control subjects. Over half of all caregivers in the study demonstrated clinically significant levels of depression. The investigators recommended that caregivers be routinely screened and, if necessary, treated by psychologists or other mental health and hospice staff.

In addition to the primary caregiver, the hospice typically forms an interdisciplinary team that can provide comprehensive care with 24-hour availability for advice or consultation. In fact, to qualify for Medicare payments, a hospice must have such a team that includes at least a physician, a registered nurse, a social worker, a chaplain, and a counselor, and it must designate a nurse to coordinate each patient's care. Most hospices employ their major team members, but hospices have a tradition of volunteerism. In fact, Medicare requires that a small percentage of hospice staff be volunteers (Field & Cassel, 1997).

The nurse and social worker typically share case management responsibilities on the hospice team. The nurse monitors the patient's physical and emotional condition. He or she educates or advises the family about how to avoid or deal with physical problems that may occur. The nurse works with physicians on the team to adjust medications as needed. He or she also develops an overall plan of care appropriate to the nature and stage of the patient's illness. The social worker, on the other hand, tends to focus on the emotional and social problems that the patient and family may encounter. He or she offers supportive counseling and functions as an advocate for both patient and family with other health care providers. The social worker also stays abreast of community resources available to terminally ill patients and advises the patient and family about how to access them.

If he or she chooses, a hospice patient may continue under the care of his or her personal physician. As the Committee on Care at the End of Life has pointed out, however, it can be difficult for a personal physician to stay involved when house calls are needed (Field & Cassel, 1997). Moreover, some physicians may not be familiar with the practices of palliative care medicine, particularly in regard to the use of opioids to relieve pain for dying patients. As mentioned earlier, many doctors remain concerned about issues of addiction and about antiaddiction laws and regulations. It may also be difficult for the personal physician to fit into a hospice team that has worked together for some time. In such instances, a hospice clinician may serve as the attending physician, but the personal physician may stay involved to provide support and information about the patient's medical history.

Although a hospice can offer many benefits to those who wish to die at home, it does not seem to have been embraced by minority populations. Thus, the Committee on Care at the End of Life has noted that more than three quarters of hospice patients are Caucasian. In part, the lack of minority use of hospice care may reflect a reluctance of minorities to abandon a curative approach to care (Caralis, Davis, Wright, & Marcial, 1993). For minorities who are enrolled in hospice care, Christakis and Iwashyna (2000) presented evidence that suggests that enrollment occurs earlier in the course of illness than for Caucasians. In fact, they noted this same trend for all disadvantaged groups in their study (i.e., minorities as well as those with lower education, lower income, psychiatric history, substance abuse history, dementia history, and advanced age). The authors argued that, in fact, this situation may be the result of stigmatized groups being seen as less appropriate for the costly, aggressive, *curative* care that is typically offered in the period preceding hospice referral.

A large percentage of hospice patients have also been reported to have received a first diagnosis of cancer. This fact is thought to reflect an emphasis by the early advocates of the hospice approach on the care of cancer patients and the provision in Medicare that death must be expected in 6 months or less for the patient to be eligible for hospice care. As noted earlier, physicians have a greater difficulty in predicting the time until death in illnesses other than cancer, and hence they are less likely to consider noncancer patients as terminal under the Medicare criteria.

Alternatives to Hospice for Home Care

Alternative arrangements for home care are important for people who don't qualify for hospice, or who are not ready to accept the assumption of the hospice program that there is no hope for a prolonged survival (Lynn, 2001). Most of these people use a mix of formal care and help from family and friends. The use of home health care agencies by Medicare beneficiaries has been increasing rapidly. These beneficiaries are typically patients with serious chronic illnesses (such as congestive heart failure) who are recognized as likely to die but not within a predictable time frame. Medicare or Medicaid certify most home health care agencies. Although the services provided by these agencies can be very helpful to seriously ill patients and their families, the Committee on End of Life Care has noted that the quality and cost-effectiveness of these services are continuing concerns (Field & Cassel, 1997). These concerns include the training and oversight of paraprofessional staff, the adequacy of attention to symptom relief, the apparently high levels of personnel turnover, and the adequacy of needs assessment and referrals to higher levels of care when required. It is thought that the quality of services provided by different home health care agencies may be quite variable, and the patient and his or her family would do well to inquire about them thoroughly and in advance.

The Committee on End of Life Care has pointed out that several HMOs have been operating their own hospices or have programs that closely parallel hospices. HMOs may actually have an incentive to encourage hospice care because Medicare picks up the end-of-life costs associated with hospices (Werth & Blevins, 2002). Although HMOs offer continuity of care, the Committee has cautioned that their staffing is likely to reflect the needs of a healthier patient population and may not match well with the needs of patients who are seriously and terminally ill. Moreover, the financial incentives that drive a managed care plan may encourage underservice to those with serious chronic illness.

Lynn (2001) has drawn attention to the gap in our home health services for those who have eventually fatal chronic illnesses but have not "transitioned to hoping only for meaningfulness and comfort" (p. 928). She has maintained that most patients nearing the end of life sometimes want and need both active treatment and comfort care. Only with the hospice program, however, does Medicare cover such palliative care. As a result, Lynn et al. (1999) proposed the creation of a new alternative Medicare supportive care benefit called *Medicaring*. Such a program would provide home care that de-emphasizes aggressive treatment, but does not make it unavailable, as is the case with hospice. Their research with focus groups has indicated that Medicaring is desired by enough people to warrant a call for demonstration programs.

A SYSTEM FOR END-OF-LIFE PREPARATION AT AN ADVANCED STAGE OF ILLNESS

Partially as a result of the Medicare criteria for terminal illnesses, hospice and palliative care have been largely limited to those who have been considered to be in their last 6 months of life. In recent years, however, efforts have been made to develop a model of psychosocial intervention that can be introduced earlier in the course of a serious disease or illness, that is, at a so-called advanced stage of illness. This model applies to those whose life expectancy due to an illness is approximately 6 to 18 months. The model is designed to supplement medical care for patients who are dying of a progressive illness but for whom death is not so near as for those considered terminal.

Approximately 2.5 million people die in the United States each year. Two million (or approximately 80%) of those who die have a protracted illness before death. Yet only about 20% of the nation's dying use hospice or palliative care, and they do so for a median time of less than 3 weeks. According to Roff and Moore (2001), several explanations can be made for this low rate of use and short length of stay: limited access to hospice and palliative care, referral criteria that require a 6-month prognosis, and referrals late in the course of the illness. The unfortunate fact is that hospice referrals are often made only when death is very close at hand. Given entry into hospice at such a late stage in the dying process, pain and symptom management usually become the major focus of care, and in actuality little time is available to address the emotional, social, and spiritual needs of the patient. Such issues have suggested a need for earlier psychosocial intervention and have given rise to a model of care alluded to earlier: the Advanced Illness Coordinated Care (AICC) model (Tobin & Larson, 2000).

Tobin (1999), who initiated the AICC model, acknowledged the many contributions of the hospice movement to care for dying patients. His position, however, has been that we need to take what hospices have done for those who are close to death and incorporate it to a greater extent at a much earlier point in the illness and dying trajectory. If work is done with patients who have advanced illnesses but are not yet terminal, there will be greater opportunity to help the patient and his or her family to understand the psychological issues involved in facing death. The goal of the work is to help the patient confront the gravity of his or her illness and begin to formulate preferences about what his or her medical care will be as the illness progresses. This approach does not rule out and, in fact, might support efforts to sustain life in situations where, for example, the patient wishes it and there is reason to try a life-prolonging or experimental treatment. It can also be used to enlighten the patient and his or her family in regard to palliative care and hospice care principles sooner than what seems to occur in our present system (Roff & Moore, 2001).

Typically, advanced illness refers to various cancer diagnoses such as cancer of the colon, liver, pancreas, and lung, as well as to diagnoses such as congestive heart failure (CHF) or chronic obstructive pulmonary disease (COPD) in which 2 or more hospitalizations or 1 or more ICU admissions have occurred within 6 months (Tobin & Larson, 2000). Central to the AICC intervention with these patients is the role of the advanced illness care coordinator. The individual filling this role typically is a nurse or a social worker, but psychologists are also qualified by their training to fulfill these functions. The case coordinator is positioned to work with the physician and the health care staff to contribute needed psychological and psychosocial support to patients and their families as the advancing illness progresses into the dying process. The physician–patient relationship remains at the center of care, but the care coordinator facilitates end-of-life conversations through a structured series of six meetings. (Although the AICC program is discussed in terms of six meetings, the number of meetings is not fixed and can be decreased or increased depending on the needs of the individual.)

In the AICC model, the initial three meetings are devoted to assessing the patient, relationship building, and setting the stage (Tobin & Larson, 2000). The first meeting is entitled *individuality and fears*. In this meeting, the care coordinator introduces himself or herself and introduces the AICC program as one that offers information and guidance to people who are facing advanced illness. The objectives are to (a) establish a collaborative relationship with the patient and family, (b) assess the patient's understanding of his or her illness, (c) assess the decision-making style of the patient and family, (d) evaluate the patient's ability to confront fears about the illness, (e) inquire about pain, and (f) inquire about advance directives and planning.

In a second meeting, entitled *fears and taking control*, the focus remains on relationship building but also on assessing the patient's major psychosocial and medical issues. Here a further approach is made toward addressing his or her fears about illness and dying. Coordinators are reminded that patients at this stage are likely to still have plans for curative treatment, and the coordinator might well support these plans. Meeting three, *practical issues*, is devoted to (a) assessing legal and social planning, (b) assessing caregiver support, (c) evaluating the patient's curative versus palliative wishes, (d) doing a more detailed evaluation of advance care planning (including an inquiry about a health care proxy), and (e) possibly planning a family meeting to discuss the patient's situation.

The second three meetings generally occur once the advanced illness has progressed and the patient is beginning to enter the dying process (Tobin & Larson, 2000). The coordinator must stay in touch with the patient and his or her family between the third and fourth meetings. The fourth meeting is a continuation of *practical issues* but, if the patient is interested, with more of a focus on palliative options and with a more aggressive assessment of advance care planning and pain management.

Meeting five is called *the turning point*. It is viewed as a pivotal phase in working with the patient whose illness is progressing. It is the point where the patient confronts the reality that he or she is dying. A shift of perspective often occurs, but cannot and should not be forced. It is an experiential shift that must be approached nondirectively using open-ended questions. The care coordinator may ask if the patient has thought about discontinuing curative efforts at care and shifting to comfort care. At such times, the patient himself or herself may begin to engage in anticipatory mourning.

In the sixth meeting, *finding peace*, the patient has presumably shifted from a cure orientation to a care orientation. It is important to confirm that the physician and the family have also made this shift. The patient may consider where he or she wishes to die and whether that be under hospice care or not. The coordinator should assure that the patient's pain and other symptoms are being assessed and treated as effectively as possible. The focus of attention changes to comfort and nurturing. The patient, if able, may want to engage in reviewing his or her life. He or she may begin to grieve and communicate feelings of loss and appreciation to family members.

Given some of the limitations in terms of access to hospice and palliative care, the AICC model seems to hold promise for assisting patients, to a greater extent than has been the case previously, in entering into the emotional and psychological work of dying with dignity. Its effectiveness has not as yet been empirically tested, but Roff and Moore (2001) indicated that a national evaluation is underway in 22 Veterans Administration (VA) and non-VA sites.

CONCLUSION

The hospice movement and its pioneers deserve great credit for having given Americans a real alternative to cure-driven conventional care at the end of life. Medicare coverage for hospice services has made that alternative a distinct possibility for many. The more complete penetration of hospice and palliative care principles into mainstream medicine and into hospitals and nursing homes, however, continues to face many challenges.

For one, it seems clearly necessary to improve efforts at educating hospital and nursing home staff in regard to the needs of dying patients and the appropriate timing and application of comfort care. Moreover, in order to enable patients to address the psychological and existential issues faced at the end of life, Medicare's 6-month criterion for entry into hospice care may need to be re-examined. Alternatively, support should be given to programs like AICC, which, prior to the final weeks of life, attempts to help patients deal with the emotional, social, and possibly spiritual issues associated with dying. Without a doubt, the underutilization of hospice care by minorities needs further investigation. In addition, laws and regulatory policies need to be shaped so that physicians can treat the pain and discomfort of dying patients without fearing that they will be accused of aiding or abetting an addiction. Finally, those who look seriously at how we die cannot help but see the great need to fund research into pain and symptom management at the end of life and, more generally, into the development of palliative medicine.

7

THE PSYCHOLOGIST'S ROLE
IN END-OF-LIFE CARE

It is one of the most difficult things in the world to do: to sit and listen while another's heart is breaking with grief, to hold the hand of a dying patient who cries silently while staring into space. . . . The very most that we can do for dying patients is to make it better, with our presence and concern, than it would be if we were not there. We can strive to facilitate emotional expression and ventilation, which have been demonstrated to be therapeutic, but we cannot "do" anything that can get rid of the psychic pain of impending loss and death.

—Rando, 1984, p. 272

Though wise men at their end know dark is right,
Because their words had forked no lightning they
Do not go gentle into that good night.

—Dylan Thomas, "Do Not Go Gentle Into That Good Night," l. 4–6[1]

As noted earlier in this book, physical pain has undeniably been a factor in the suffering experienced by many dying patients. Nonetheless, studies
have indicated that psychological pain and psychosocial distress (e.g., loss of
dignity, feelings of dependency, fears of disintegration, and loss of community)

have been the major contributing factors for those dying patients who have felt that assisted suicide or euthanasia might be their best option (Lavery, Boyle, Dickens, MacLean, & Singer, 2001; van der Maas, van Delden, Pijnenborg, & Looman, 1991). The findings in these studies leave little doubt about the need for psychological assistance and efforts at psychosocial intervention with the dying patient. Consistent with hospice and palliative care principles, the general objectives for psychologists are to assist the terminally ill patient in living as fully and as comfortably as possible during the so-called *living-dying interval*. The objectives also include helping the patient and his or her family prepare for the patient's eventual death (Rando, 1984).

Helping the patient and his or her family prepare for death does not necessarily mean that the psychologist expects the patient to reach an acceptance of death. As Rando (1984) pointed out, many question the goal of facilitating an acceptance of death and wonder if the notion has been promoted more for those who must witness death than for the actual patient. In Rando's experience, true acceptance is seldom realized, yet that does not mean that a so-called *good death* cannot be achieved. Although the patient may fight against dying, what eventually seems to occur is more of a realization that death is inevitable. Caregivers, and particularly psychologists, can help the patient during this time of struggle by helping him or her to retain as much control, dignity, and self-esteem as possible, but perhaps it is better that some resistance to dying be maintained than that all hope be abandoned.

As members of the American Psychological Association's (APA's) Ad Hoc Committee on End-of-Life Issues, Haley, Neimeyer, Larson, Kwilosz, and Kasl-Godley (2003) articulated four time periods when psychologists might be involved in end-of-life care: (a) before life-threatening illness strikes, (b) during the period of advanced illness, (c) during terminal illness, and (d) during the period of bereavement following death. In the present chapter , we examine the possible roles and functions that mental health clinicians, particularly psychologists, might have during each of these time periods. In addition, we discuss the possible roles of psychologists in the hospice and palliative care systems as well as their roles as members of Ethics Advisory Committees (EACs).

PRIOR TO A PROGRESSIVE AND LIFE-THREATENING ILLNESS

With regard to patients who have not yet developed a life-threatening illness, a great need seems to exist for psychologists to help prepare these patients for the time when a serious illness may strike. Such an involvement is particularly appropriate for those patients who are aging and may be at a heightened risk for chronic and progressive illnesses. In chapter 3 of this book, we discuss advance care planning and some of the difficulties that have been encountered in attempting to implement it (e.g., The SUPPORT Principal Investigators, 1995). One of the chapter's conclusions is that the importance of both the patient–clinician relationship and good communication tends to be overlooked in the standard and formulaic approach to the completion of advance directives. In fact, Tulsky, Fischer, Rose, and Arnold (1998) found that physicians in their study spent a median of 5.6 minutes in their discussions of advance directives with patients, and, of that total time, the patient had an average of 2 minutes to speak. The physicians in this study were found to focus on whether the patient wanted specific interventions rather than on an exploration of the reasons for the patient's preferences and values.

In both the Lacrosse Advance Directive Study (LADS; Hammes & Rooney, 1998) and in the Molloy et al. (2000) study in Canada, greater success with advance care planning was reported. Both of these studies employed extensive advance directive education programs (the *Respecting Your Choices* and the *Let Me Decide* programs respectively). They also viewed advance care planning as an ongoing process and shifted the focus of discussion away from completing a form or document to a discussion of values and preferences. The investigators used nonphysician advance directive educators who were available and accessible to staff and patients.

With their emphasis on interpersonal sensitivity and good communication skills, psychologists (e.g., those in behavioral medicine or gerontology) seem very suited to this type of process-oriented discussion. They also seem more inclined to encourage the use of some of the newer, more personalized living will and health care proxy documents, such as the *Five Wishes* (Commission on Aging with Dignity, 1998) and the *Your Life, Your Choices* (Pearlman et al., 2001) documents.

Given that community education programs about advance care planning have been helpful, there would seem to be a role for psychologists in this type of activity. In fact, Haley et al. (2003) highlighted one such innovative effort called *Finding Our Way: Living with Dying in America*, a 15-article newspaper series on end-of-life issues, with a psychologist as senior editor (Larson, 2001). This series contains articles by experts on not only advance directives but also topics such as caregiving, hospice, palliative care, the death of children, widowhood, and so forth. It is replete with the stories of real people who have struggled with these end-of-life issues. It provides information on resources for the dying patient and his or her family, and in so doing, the series attempts to combat the sense of helplessness and loss of control so frequently encountered by terminally ill patients. Hopefully, other psychologists can take this publication as an impetus to develop other end-of-life psychoeducational programs and resource guides.

DURING THE PERIOD OF ADVANCED ILLNESS

As Haley et al. (2003) pointed out, a comprehensive approach to care calls attention to the needs of patients and their families throughout the course of their illness. The period of prolonged and advanced illness can provide many opportunities for the psychologist to make positive contributions to the care of the patient and his or her family. Perhaps he or she can be most effective as part of an interdisciplinary health care team. Currently, some experimentation is taking place in clinical settings with a variety of different teams; a hospice consultation team, a symptom control team, an advanced illness coordinated care team (Tobin & Larson, 2000), and so forth. The purpose of these teams is to work with the patient population that is suffering with a prolonged illness and to identify medical, psychological, and psychosocial problems that they might help to resolve. These teams can also facilitate the overall coordination of care.

Of course, one of the major psychological or emotional problems in a medically ill population is depression. As Cassem (1995) noted, the rates of major depression rise when a serious medical illness is present. Elderly patients in outpatient primary care settings have rates of depression ranging from 2.7% to 8.6%, while community-dwelling elders have rates of only 1% (Coyne, Fechner-Bates, & Schwenk, 1994; Schade, Jones, & Wittlin, 1998). The rates of major depression in elderly patients hospitalized because of a medical illness have been found to be over 10 times that reported in the community (Koenig & Blazer, 1992). In a study of 3 U.S. sites involving 11,242 outpatients, Wells, Golding, and Burnam (1988) noted that depression and medical conditions had unique and additive effects on patient functioning. The combination of depression and current advanced coronary artery disease was associated with roughly twice the reduction in social functioning (e.g., visiting with family and friends, going to social activities) as that which occurs in either condition alone. Cole and Bellevance (1997), in a meta-analysis of eight studies, found that elderly medical inpatients who were depressed had significantly higher mortality rates than elderly patients in hospital-based psychiatric services. It is known, however, that physicians often fail to detect depression in the medically ill, or they view it as "appropriate" to the patient's condition (Cassem, 1995; Rihmer, Rutz, & Pihlgren, 1995). In fact, after a review of the literature on this topic, Peruzzi, Canapary, and Bongar (1996) concluded that "the capacity of physicians untrained in psychiatry to diagnose depression (was) alarmingly low" (p. 354). Depression thus frequently goes untreated in a medical population.

Block (2000) has made efforts to assist physicians and others in distinguishing depression from the normal grief and distress encountered among terminally ill patients. Thus, she proposed that a number of differences be noted, such as (a) a depressed patient is anhedonic while the grieving or distressed patient retains some capacity for pleasure; (b) depression is constant, while grief and distress tend to come in waves; and (c) depressed patients have no sense of a positive future, while distressed patients can still, at times, look to the future. These distinctions seem very useful clinically and it is hoped that they will be studied further.

The fact that physicians generally undertreat depression in the medically ill led the Swedish Committee for Prevention and Treatment of Depression to introduce a trial educational program for all general practitioners on the island of Gotland (pop. 56,000). As Rutz, von Knorring, and Walinder (1989) stated, the primary goal of this program was to increase knowledge about the diagnosis and treatment of patients with affective disorders. The educational effort consisted of two 2-day programs to which all general practitioners were invited, and about 90% attended. The programs included lectures on the classification, etiology, and pathogenesis of depressive disorders; treating depressed patients; depressive disorders in old age; and so forth. The study found that, during the year after the educational program, significantly more patients with depressive disorders were identified and treated adequately than during the prior year. The suicide rate on Gotland also dropped significantly, both relative to the rate for Gotland and to the rate for Sweden as a whole. In fact, the year following the educational program was the only year in a 17-year period in which there was a significant difference in the suicide rate between Gotland and Sweden as a whole.

Findings such as these seem to lend emphasis to the importance of having a psychologist on an interdisciplinary team in order to offer consultations about patients with advanced and progressive illnesses. A three-year follow-up to the Gotland study found that the positive effects of the educational program had not lasted (Rutz, von Knorring, & Walinder, 1992). The authors concluded that the program had a pronounced effect, but it was related in time strictly to the educational effort. They suggested that if a long term effect is to be achieved, the educational program would need to be repeated about every two years. With a psychologist as a regular member of an advanced illness consultation team, however, heightened awareness of and education about emotional disorders in the medically ill can be ongoing.

Depression, as noted earlier, is not the only emotional problem encountered by those with serious medical illnesses. Many also suffer with anxiety, fear of a painful death, fear of abandonment, sadness, and a sense of loss. These problems can often be diminished by a combination of supportive psychotherapy, training in various coping skills (e.g., relaxation techniques, the use of imagery, and skills in setting priorities), and medications. In addition, the patient's family can, at times, be enlisted to assist the patient in his or her efforts to cope. If the goal is to introduce principles of palliative care and improve the quality of life for those with advanced but not yet terminal conditions, then, as Haley et al. (2003) stated, "the best way to achieve this goal is to integrate medical and psychological symptom management, psychosocial support, and advance care planning" (p. 9).

Of course, chronic pain is another frequent problem for patients with many advanced and progressive illnesses. Medical, pharmacological, and surgical interventions are often only partially successful in alleviating such pain. Hence, Turk and Okifuji (2002) suggested a biopsychosocial model (rather than a biomedical model) of pain in which the individual's response to pain is shaped by the interaction of biological, psychological, and sociocultural factors. This model has been instrumental in the development of behavioral and cognitive–behavioral treatments for pain. In this regard, McCracken and Turk (2002), in a meta-analytic review of controlled studies, reported evidence that treatments of this sort have been effective for some patients in decreasing (although not eliminating) pain, reducing emotional distress related to pain, and improving the ability to cope with and accept pain. Generally, those who perceive some ability to control their pain have been found to benefit more from behavioral and cognitive–behavioral treatment. In any event, psychologists could clearly add nonpharmacological pain management techniques to the armamentarium of interdisciplinary teams working with patients for whom chronic pain is an issue. Simon and Folen (2001) described how such a role can effectively be established.

WHEN THE PATIENT'S CONDITION IS CONSIDERED TERMINAL

One is reminded that the boundary between what have been referred to as advanced illness and terminal illness can be very difficult to determine. No known cure exists for conditions like congestive heart failure or chronic obstructive pulmonary disease, but patients can live with them for years. The Committee on Care at the End of Life (Field & Cassel, 1997) has spoken of the great uncertainty in predicting life expectancy with such illnesses. In effect, we consider an illness as terminal when the prevailing medical opinion is that the patient is gravely ill, that the end is approaching, and that he or she seems unlikely to be able to sustain life beyond the next several months to a year. There is little certainty about when a patient crosses this line.

As with the patient with advanced illness, the psychologist who wishes to work with the terminally ill can probably be most effective as part of an interdisciplinary team. Hospice and palliative care programs are generally organized according to an interdisciplinary team concept. The hospice philosophy is to treat the person, not the disease; and, hence, medical services are only a part of the approach to care (Marwit, 1997).

Despite the team model in hospices, however, at least one of the mental health disciplines, psychology, has been virtually absent from the list of core hospice service providers (Hartman-Stein, 2001). The roots of this issue remain unclear, but the APA's recently appointed Ad Hoc Committee on End-of-Life Issues has noted that psychology as a field has either overlooked, or perhaps avoided, an area of practice where it has much to contribute (DeAngelis, 2002). The question now is whether psychologists have been locked out, so to speak, because there is a long established core hospice team that already includes other mental health disciplines or because of complicated reimbursement regulations. This would be unfortunate because the need for psychological services in this area of practice is only likely to increase as the baby boomer generation ages and must confront the deaths of parents and their own mortality. Clearly, efforts need to be made to increase the involvement of professional psychology in hospice and palliative care team functions.

The Psychologist's Role in Evaluation and Intervention

Among the mental health disciplines, psychology has demonstrated great strength in the development and use of standardized assessment instruments. Currently, several instruments with good psychometric properties are being used to assess death-related issues (Neimeyer & Van Brunt, 1995). These scales and questionnaires assess attitudes toward death, the variations of death anxiety, and death acceptance or avoidance. They can be used not only as clinical and research instruments but also as informal guides to the evaluation of patient concerns about dying.

Good evaluation and identification of problems leads to appropriate intervention. As in the case of advanced illnesses, those with terminal illness typically have a number of psychological and psychosocial issues that are amenable to intervention. Many of the terminally ill have treatable depression, anxiety, pain, and fear, as well as existential concerns about dying that can be alleviated to a degree. Thus, Chochinov, Wilson, Enns, and Lander (1998) found that hopelessness was an important clinical marker for suicidal ideation in dying patients, and Breitbart et al. (2000) found that depression and hopelessness were the strongest predictors of the desire for a hastened death in their sample of terminally ill cancer patients. In the study by Breitbart et al., patients who were neither depressed nor hopeless did not have a desire for hastened death. Many patients in this study were able to maintain hope even in the final weeks of life, although what they hoped for changed. Those terminally ill patients who are depressed and hopeless may be amenable to psychological interventions, although it will be important to identify those treatments that can be empirically shown to be of value.

Aside from falling victim to depression and hopelessness, terminally ill patients typically have many concerns about death and dying, and counselors can assist them in dealing with these issues. As Chochinov (2000) highlighted, patients often have questions and fears about the suffering they may have to endure or the bodily changes and disfigurement that will occur. They may be concerned about abandonment because of the negative changes in their ability to function and in their appearance. They sometimes search for continued purpose and meaning as they confront death, and they may fear loss of independence and control. These are issues that a good psychotherapist or counselor is trained to understand, and in the face of them, he or she can help the patient to cope and to achieve some comfort.

At times, patients will seek assistance with difficult decisions about whether to abandon curative efforts for comfort care, or whether to pursue a course that will have a secondary effect of hastening death. In this regard, Goldblum and Martin (1999) proposed a collaborative decision-making model and posed a series of questions that might provide guidance to the psychologist or mental health practitioner working with patients who are confronting such issues.

In this model, a negative answer to any of the following questions would suggest that the patient should not be encouraged or permitted to pursue a decision that may not continue to sustain life. First, does the patient perceive his or her condition to be unbearable? Second, is the patient receiving adequate medical care (including comfort care)? Third, does the patient understand his or her condition, prognosis, and treatment options? Fourth, is the patient's thinking free of psychologically based distortion? Fifth, does the patient have adequate social support and have his or her significant others been involved in the discussion? Finally, has the patient clearly and repeatedly expressed the desire to die? If the answer to all these questions is affirmative, then a decision to withdraw or withhold life-sustaining treatment, or a decision that might have the double effect of hastening death, would seem to be acceptable.

If a patient is considering assisted suicide (as in Oregon where it is legal), Werth (1999b) and Werth, Benjamin, and Farrenkopf (2000) proposed detailed guidelines with which the psychologist should be familiar. In discussing such questions, however, the clinician will need to make it clear that providing or delivering a means to end life is definitely outside the scope of practice for psychologists and other nonmedical treatment providers.

The family is a key component in work with the dying patient, yet family members are also very stressed by the loss they are experiencing and the caregiving they must provide. Rando (1986) referred to family members as "the commonly overlooked secondary victims of terminal illness" (p. 99) who must witness the progressive debilitation of their loved ones. The patient's decline often is characterized by many ups and downs requiring many adaptations and readaptations, and the emotional toll can be heavy on family members. As noted in chapter 6, the terminally ill patient who is cared for at home usually needs extensive assistance from the family (Emanuel et al., 1999). If a hospice program is involved, they often require that a family member be designated as primary caregiver. These individuals carry a substantial burden for the patient and the family. Although further research on this topic is needed, Haley et al. (2003) have indicated that family caregivers appear to have a higher incidence of depression than noncaregiving controls. Moreover, Marwit (1997) argued that there is an increased mortality for surviving spouses (and possibly other family members) within the first 6 months after a death in the family. Thus, one needs to be concerned not only with the health needs of the dying patient but also with the health needs of family members.

The psychologist on a hospice or palliative care team would be well suited to provide support and intervention for stressed family members. Although little research has been done on the effectiveness of interventions with family members who help with end-of-life care, the National Hospice Study found that primary caregivers working with the support of a hospice were more satisfied with the patients' care than their counterparts working in a conventional care system (Greer et al., 1986). Hospices are also committed to bereavement follow-up and counseling, something that is not typically found in conventional care. Intervention with the distressed or grieving family or family member appears to be another area where the psychologist can make a significant difference, and, of course, he or she can engage in these clinical efforts as well as in conducting research to investigate which interventions can be, in some measure, validated.

The Psychologist's Role as Consultant on Decision Making

As terminally ill patients become more debilitated, questions about their capacity to make health care decisions are not uncommon. Some of these decisions, such as those that have implications in terms of hastening death, have obviously serious consequences. The criteria and methods for making determinations of a patient's decision-making capacity or incapacity are discussed in chapter 2. For the patient who does not have a history that is complicated by mental illness or cognitive impairment, it is often the attending physician who makes this determination and also decides whether reason exists to pursue having a surrogate decision maker designated for the patient. If the case is complicated by the presence of a mental or emotional disorder, however, the health care system typically requires that a licensed psychologist or a psychiatrist be consulted to evaluate the patient's capacity for decision making. In regard to who is authorized to conduct such evaluations, the individual practitioner is advised to check the policy of the health care system or institution for whom he or she works.

Those psychologists and psychiatrists who take on this consulting role need to be well versed in the relevant ethical and forensic issues involved. A patient's capacity or incapacity for making health care decisions is usually determined after a review of the medical records, discussions with staff and the patient's family (if appropriate), and an interview with the patient. Often, it is important to have the attending physician or his designee accompany the consultant and describe the patient's condition and any proposed treatment in plain language. The consultant can then question the patient about his or her understanding of the issues. With particularly complicated cases, it may also be an aid to the evaluator to use a standardized assessment instrument like the MacArthur Competence Assessment Tool for Treatment Decisions (MacCAT-T; Grisso & Appelbaum, 1998). Given their background in assessment, psychologists are best suited for administering and interpreting such instruments.

The Psychologist's Role in Assisting Staff With the Stress of End-of-Life Care

Caring for the dying patient can be stressful for family members as well as for staff who work in hospice, palliative care, nursing home, or hospital settings. Although they may not have as extensive or intensive a relationship with the patient as a family member, staff members form an emotional attachment to their patients. It is often difficult for them to witness the dying process in a patient for whom they have provided care for a long time. If they have had a romanticized view of the *good death*, they may become disillusioned as they see the reality of the suffering associated with most deaths. As Rando (1984) noted, working with the patient who is on a trajectory towards death can be a threat to the staff's sense of mastery and control. When staff repeatedly feel helpless and stressed, they can become vulnerable to emotional and physical exhaustion or *burnout*. In addition, work with dying patients can bring up personal issues for staff members. These can include a heightened awareness of their own past losses, increased concern about likely future family losses, and increased anxiety about their own mortality.

Given the emotional challenges that confront staff members in this type of work, it is very important to ensure that support and resources for assistance are available. In a team-oriented setting, psychologists are ideally suited to encourage and facilitate regular group support meetings that are focused on the needs of the staff caregivers. Sharing feelings of sadness, loss, frustration, and anger with peers who understand and who may be experiencing the same emotions can be very helpful in maintaining stability. If a patient dies, the psychologist can facilitate a closure meeting at which staff can review their feelings about the loss and remember the deceased. The demands of working with death and dying need to be continuously recognized by staff and by their supervisors. If individual staff members are particularly distressed, a psychologist should be accessible for counseling or therapeutic intervention.

The Psychologist's Role in Research on Death and Dying

In recent years, the discipline of psychology has taken a renewed pride in its training in, and emphasis on research and evidence-based practices. In the study of death and dying, its academic and research activity has been voluminous (see, e.g., the review by Niemeyer & van Brunt, 1995). As Niemeyer and van Brunt noted, however, much of this past research has lacked relevance to the real-life problems encountered by the patient who is experiencing the living-with-dying process.

Psychology clearly needs to direct more research effort to assessing the psychosocial needs of terminally ill patients and their families, as well as to studying psychological and behavioral interventions that may prove helpful in meeting those needs. In addition, further research on the psychological and psychosocial factors that contribute to patients' requests to hasten death will be very important. As Rosenfeld (2000) pointed out, research with terminally ill patients is complicated by a number of factors, not the least of which is the frequent incidence of cognitive impairment that occurs as terminal illness advances. He has stressed, however, the importance of attempting to work longitudinally with those patients who progress to the late stages of disease but without significant cognitive deterioration. These patients are likely to be involved in making the relevant decisions about whether to attempt to prolong their lives or not. Among the mental health disciplines, psychology, in collaboration with neuropsychology, has the capabilities to assess these patients and attempt such complicated and challenging research.

DURING THE PERIOD OF BEREAVEMENT

One of the very good aspects of the hospice program for end-of-life care is that family members are offered bereavement counseling after the patient's death. Psychologists clearly have a role in providing such services. One should not assume, however, that because these services are provided after the death of the patient that they are meant to imply that assistance with grief and mourning begins with the patient's death. Whether one subscribes to the idea of *anticipatory mourning* or not, most thanatologists agree that certain preparations for loss often occur during the period in which the patient is dying, especially when this period is prolonged as in most modern deaths (Rando, 1986; 2000). Moreover, smaller losses occur during the living–dying period that often evoke lower levels of grief than are found in the actual death of a loved one. Thus, one may experience grief at seeing the loss of the loved one's health, ability to function, ability to relate, and the promise of a future together. Family and friends can often use the support and therapeutic intervention of a counselor to facilitate coping with these more subtle and less tangible losses that precede death.

Thanatologists have noted that, once death has occurred, several tasks or processes of mourning need to be completed if the surviving family and friends are to re-establish an emotional equilibrium and go on living. Worden (1991), for example, referred to four tasks of mourning: (a) to accept the reality of the loss, (b) to work through the pain and grief, (c) to adjust to an environment in which the deceased is missing, and (d) to emotionally relocate the deceased and move on with life. He used the term *relocate* in recognition of the fact that the bereaved never completely give up their relationship to the deceased. Rather, they need to find a place for the dead in their emotional lives that allows them to invest in other people and move on with living. Rando (1995), similarly, wrote of *the six R processes* of mourning. These consist of the following: (a) recognizing the loss, (b) reacting to the separation (or experiencing the pain), (c) recollecting and re-experiencing the deceased and the relationship (this includes remembering both positive and negative feelings toward the deceased), (d) relinquishing the old attachments to the deceased and the old assumptive world, (e) readjusting to move adaptively into the new world without forgetting the old, and (f) reinvesting emotional energy into new attachments.

In negotiating such a mourning process, several forms of counseling and assistance are typically available to those who wish to use them (Worden, 1991). First, one can join a self-help group in which an individual who has suffered a loss meets with others who have also experienced losses. These groups provide the person with an opportunity to share feelings and experiences related to the death of a loved one, and to learn how others have coped in the wake of losing a significant other. Second, there are some bereavement counseling services in which volunteer counselors have been trained and supported by professionals. These may be widow-to-widow programs or their equivalent (depending on the relationship of the bereaved to the deceased). Finally, there are grief counseling and therapy services provided by mental health professionals. These services are usually offered on either an individual basis or in a group setting with others who have struggled with a significant loss.

Loss and grief are an inevitable part of the human experience. Most people suffer with losses, go through the several phases of mourning, obtain support from family and friends, allow their attachment to the deceased to diminish, and, within 4 to 6 months, show significant signs of adjusting to their changed world. Others, however, may actually be subject to an increased risk of illness and even mortality after bereavement. Thus, Kaprio, Koskenvuo, and Rita (1987) did a linkage study with over 95,000 widowed persons in Finland and found a significantly increased risk of death from ischemic heart disease for both men and women in the first week after a spouse's death. During the first month of widowhood, these same authors also reported a 17-fold increase in death by suicide for men and a 4.5-fold increase in death by suicide for women. Still others may not be subject to illness or death, but may have difficulty grieving or be unable to complete the grieving process or develop complications like prolonged and intense grief reactions. Such individuals (who are said to have complicated bereavement or pathological grief) are very likely to need the assistance of a mental health professional who is trained to work with such conditions.

In work with the family and friends of the dying patient, the mental health practitioner can use his or her expertise to identify those family members who are most likely to be at risk of having greater difficulty with bereavement. Rando (1995) delineated several factors thought to be associated with subsequent complications in the mourning process. These include (a) a markedly angry, ambivalent, or dependent relationship to the dying patient; (b) prior difficulties with losses; (c) concurrent mental health problems; and (d) a perceived lack of social support. She also noted that specific types of death may be likely to precipitate difficulties with mourning, such as the death of a child, a death that was seen as preventable, or death that was either unanticipated and sudden or due to an overly lengthy illness.

In an interesting recent investigation, Prigerson et al. (1997) presented evidence indicating that grief and depression declined steeply for most of their subjects within the first 6 months after a loss. If, after 6 months, however, significant symptoms of what the authors referred to as *traumatic* or complicated grief were still present, they were found to be predictive of traumatic or complicated grief at 1 year and 2 years after the loss. The investigators conceptualized traumatic grief as related to trauma and separation distress, and consisting of ongoing symptoms such as feeling disbelief and shock about the death, being preoccupied with thoughts of the deceased, yearning and searching for the deceased, having survival guilt over the death, and so forth. If clinicians are sensitive to and able to track these types of reactions closely, therapeutic interventions that may prevent more chronic grief reactions can be suggested and initiated.

Much has been written about therapies for unresolved or complicated grief (e.g., Niemeyer, 2001; Rando, 1984; Worden, 1991). Unfortunately, we have little data on which of these therapies are effective and for whom. In a meta-analysis of the effectiveness of grief therapy, Allumbaugh and Hoyt (1999) found equivocal outcomes for much of grief counseling and therapy. Interestingly, however, in a small number of studies, they found that grief therapy had a strong positive effect with self-selected clients. Thus, bereaved individuals who voluntarily sought treatment appeared to benefit more than those who were recruited for treatment studies. The authors hypothesized that those who sought treatment may have had higher initial distress levels and hence more potential for improvement. They also felt that it was reasonable to believe that they were more highly motivated than those agreeing to treatment because of a research team's recruiting efforts. As with other forms of psychotherapy, motivation looms large as a determinant of successful outcome with grief therapy.

THE PSYCHOLOGIST AND END-OF-LIFE INTERDISCIPLINARY TEAMS AND COMMITTEES

Psychologists who work in hospitals and clinics have a long history of functioning as members of multidisciplinary treatment teams. Their skills in collaborative work seem readily transferrable to end-of-life practices. As noted earlier, terminally ill patients and their families face a multitude of psychological and psychosocial issues. They need the availability and expertise that can be provided by different mental health disciplines.

Because the potential contributions of psychologists to hospice and palliative care teams have been articulated throughout the preceding sections of this chapter, we will not reiterate them here. Suffice it to say that the approaches and values espoused in hospice and palliative care settings are quite compatible with the orientation of mental health clinicians such as psychologists. As DeAngelis (2002) pointed out, the hospice emphasis on the holistic needs of the patient, as well as on work with the families of patients, are aspects of care in which psychologists are generally well versed. Psychologists with expertise in gerontology and behavioral medicine have particular skills to bring to the dying patient and to the end-of-life care team. These include not only skills in therapeutic intervention and the assessment of mood and anxiety disorders in an elderly and medically ill population, but also specific techniques that can be useful in pain and stress management. In addition, psychologists can be available to help families whose emotional distress may be beyond what frontline clinical staff, who are occupied with nursing or medical duties, can manage.

The remainder of this section will be devoted to discussing another form of collaborative involvement for psychologists interested in end-of-life issues. Most hospitals and health care systems today have an ethics advisory committee (EAC) that is interdisciplinary in its composition. These committees are actually of relatively recent origin, having been first strongly encouraged by the President's Commission for the Study of Ethical Problems in Medicine and Biomedical and Behavioral Research (1983). They have become extremely important committees in terms of dealing with complicated end-of-life cases and issues. Membership on such a committee typically includes professional care providers from a wide range of disciplines. Actually, EAC membership is intended to reflect the professional composition of the institution.

There has been a good deal of discussion of, but no consensus on, the knowledge base and skills that EAC members should possess. The American Society for Bioethics and Humanities (1998) issued a report on core competencies for health care ethics consultation. In terms of knowledge, the Society has recommended that, among other things, EAC members have a basic understanding of moral reasoning and ethical theory, as well as of the bioethical concepts that are typically employed in ethics consultations. They have maintained that basic skills should include ethical assessment skills (or an ability to identify underlying value conflicts and uncertainties), process skills (or an ability to facilitate the resolution of value conflicts), and interpersonal skills (or an ability to listen well, communicate effectively, and elicit as well as represent the views of others). The Society has suggested a variety of ways in which EAC members may acquire basic ethical knowledge and skill. These include taking basic courses, completing independent study courses, attending education programs and conferences, and pursuing self-education.

In general, EACs provide a forum for the discussion of ethical issues that arise in patient care. The presence of an ethics committee contributes to the institution by encouraging clinicians and the health care system itself to carry on evaluations of how they function in activities that have an ethical dimension. It is also hoped that the EAC will provide a process for resolving disputes about treatment. In so doing, some have hoped that it might decrease the likelihood of institutional and individual liability (VA National Headquarters Bioethics Committee, 1996), while others have been concerned that such a focus (on liability control) will give the committee a risk management orientation and undermine its ethical purposes (Annas, 1991). If EACs remain aware of such possibilities, however, they need not be co-opted by the needs of the institution in this regard. Needless to say, the participation of psychologists on an EAC is crucial in terms of heightening recognition of the many psychological and psychosocial issues that have ethical implications in end-of-life decision making.

EACs have several functions. First, they educate clinical staff, patients, and their families. In this regard, they attempt to foster an ethically knowledgeable and sensitive health care system where there can be a constructive discussion about ethical issues and dilemmas. Ethics education can be promoted through presentations at meetings such as Grand Rounds and at EAC-sponsored conferences and workshops. Information about ethical issues can be conveyed to patients and families on posters, in pamphlets, and in patient handbooks covering topics such as patients' rights, advance care planning, or informed consent.

Second, EACs serve a case consultation function. Patients, surrogates, and all members of the clinical staff have the right to initiate a request for an ethics consultation. Typically, a small EAC subcommittee will be designated to respond to specific consultation requests. The subcommittee reviews the clinical record and meets with the treatment team as well as with the patient with or without his or her family as indicated. At times, the process of consulting may lead to a resolution of the conflict, or the subcommittee may advise the parties involved to attempt to pursue other avenues that might lead to a resolution. In any event, the subcommittee will offer recommendations based on an application of ethical principles to the issues raised. These recommendations are considered advisory in nature, and the final decision ultimately remains with the responsible clinical team members. Instances can occur, however, when the EAC or its subcommittee feels that important rights are in jeopardy. After efforts to resolve the issue have been made, the EAC might report its findings and recommendations to someone like the chief of service or the chief of staff who has the authority to ensure a fair and just outcome. Psychologists, with their skill in conflict management, can be important members of the consultation team. Moreover, many EACs require the participation of a psychologist or psychiatrist if the issue involves a patient who has a history of mental illness.

The EAC has a third role, which is to review and offer direction for institutional policies that have definite ethical implications. Thus, for example, the EAC is typically consulted in the development of policies on advance care planning, informed consent, withholding and withdrawing life-sustaining treatment, palliative care, and so forth. Once again, the committee's role is advisory, but it can ensure that ethical considerations are taken into account in the policies that govern patient care, particularly end-of-life care.

Finally, the EAC has a role to play in encouraging quality assurance reviews as well as research and scholarly inquiry into areas of clinical ethics and organizational ethics. Mental health practitioners such as psychologists, who often have a research background, can be instrumental in promoting such evaluative and empirical efforts. As the APA Working Group on Assisted Suicide and End-of-Life Decisions (2000) pointed out, the quality and amount of research on end-of-life decision making is limited. Clearly, a need exists for further research on topics like optimal end-of-life experiences, the adequacy of palliative care, the effect of caregiver burden on end-of-life decisions, and the availability and quality of psychological services for terminally ill patients and their families.

CONCLUSION

In this chapter, we have reviewed the many roles and functions that psychologists can fulfill in end-of-life care. Although disciplines like psychiatry and clinical social work may not be totally satisfied with their participation in this area of practice (see, e.g., Cochinov, 2000), psychology as a discipline has been particularly invisible in professional discussions of end-of-life issues and in clinical activity with the dying patient (Working Group, 2000). That is not to say that individual psychologists have not made significant contributions. The APA Working Group, however, was formed to make recommendations that might bring psychology as a discipline into the national discourse on end-of-life care. It is, after all, difficult to conceive of a more intensely emotional and psychological time than when a patient is facing his or her decline and eventual death. Surely psychologists, in collaboration with their colleagues from other health and mental health disciplines, have much to offer dying patients, their families, and those who bear the burden of care giving.

8

CONCLUDING THOUGHTS ON
SUFFERING, DYING, AND CHOICE

What I hope, unfortunately, is not what I expect. I have seen too much of death to ignore the overwhelming odds that it will not occur as I wish it. Like most people, I will probably suffer with the physical and emotional distress that accompany many mortal illnesses, and like most people I will probably compound the pained uncertainty of my last months by the further agony of indecision—to continue or to give in, to be treated aggressively or to be comforted, to struggle for the possibility of more time or to call it a day and a life . . .

—Nuland, 1993, pp. 263–264

Despite great advances in the management of physical pain, few people who die of progressive illnesses go through them without suffering. As Byock (1996) maintained, physical pain is insufficient to explain or account for suffering (a term that has psychological and emotional meaning), yet in medical circles suffering is often understood only in terms of physical pain. Cassel (1982) attributed medicine's relatively exclusive focus on physical pain to the mind–body dichotomy introduced into Western philosophical thought by René Descartes. In asserting a split between mind and body, the body and its functions historically became the domain of science and medicine, while the mind and spirit remained in the realm of the church. As Cassel pointed out, however, it is a *person* who suffers, not simply a body. It is the person, with all of his or her individual characteristics and life experiences, who feels that his or her integrity is threatened, or that he or she is diminished, by injury or disease. From this perspective, Western medicine has had too narrow a focus to deal with what is implied in the term *suffering*. An exclusive emphasis on the cure of bodily disease, however, has led to the conditions where physicians, at times, have done things to combat disease that in the larger picture cause suffering for individuals.

Yet even in the realm of the physical, some forms of distress are difficult to alleviate or manage. Take the AIDS patient, for example, who may suffer with symptoms of fever, night sweats, fatigue, diarrhea, anemia, nausea, vomiting, draining sores, sore throat, gastrointestinal ulcerations, mental confusion, and so forth (Nuland, 1993). Decreasing or eliminating pain will not necessarily do away with such forms of physical distress or, for that matter, with suffering. For suffering is psychological in nature and is more related to the loss of meaning and purpose in life, or, as noted earlier, to the individual's awareness of his or her disintegration as a functioning being (Byock, 1996; Cassel, 1982; Rando, 1984).

In spite of such suffering, there are, nonetheless, many who have espoused the notion that *good* or *peaceful* dying is attainable if we approach the dying process in the proper way. Block (2001) and Byock (1996), for example, have spoken of the opportunities for transformation or transcendence during the dying process. They have cited anecdotal evidence of those who have resolved long-standing family conflicts, or who learned to be more understanding and compassionate while dying, or who even became mentors to their care providers. Tobin (1999) has also written of transforming the dying process "from a process of fear to one of jubilation" (p. 154) by focusing on the loving relationships in one's life as well as on spirituality.

Little doubt exists that such transformations are occasionally observed; however, if not balanced against the painful realities of so many deaths, the approaches above would seem to be at great risk of contributing to the mythology that dying typically occurs in a state of tranquility with one's loved ones gathered about for a final, deeply felt farewell. With such illusory images of dying, we can allay our fear and repugnance of death, but we also compromise our ability to prepare for what is likely to come. Byock (1996) noted that the frequency of such transforming experiences is not known. Certainly, they are difficult to imagine with patients who have Alzheimer's disease or Parkinson's disease or who are so distressed with dyspnea and end-stage chronic obstructive pulmonary disease (COPD) that they can focus on little beyond their next breath. Rather, the norm seems more akin to the description given by Rando (1984), "For death, in far too many cases, is not romantic. It is not graceful. It is not beautiful. In fact, death stinks—literally and figuratively! It is clammy, too. It can sound bad, and it often is ugly" (p. 272).

Nuland (1993), among others, has written of the need to demythologize the process of dying so that patients will be less subject to self-deception and disillusionment at life's end. Perhaps a more realistic approach to what can be expected in the dying process has been captured in the term coined by Battin (1994), "the least worst death" (p. 36). Given that a phrase like *good death* or *dying well* sounds somewhat like an oxymoron, or at least seems unattainable for many, *the least worst death* among those that might conceivably occur for a particular individual seems more reality based. In attempting to bring about the least worst death, the physician and the entire treatment team, in collaboration with the patient and his or her family, become strategists for how the patient might meet death most favorably and with the fewest negative experiences.

Whether it be acute or long-term terminal illness, Battin (1994) pointed out that the key to a good strategy for achieving the least worst death is flexibility in considering all the options. In this regard, the treatment team respects the patient's autonomy and right to self-determination by providing him or her with information about the risks and benefits of all the possible courses of action, not simply information related to a choice between accepting or refusing a single procedure favored by the staff. For example, if a patient has cancer of the bowel that could cause an obstruction and he or she also has a serious infection, the patient would need to know the likely consequences of (a) accepting bowel surgery and antibiotics, (b) taking antibiotics with no immediate surgery, (c) having surgery with no antibiotics, or (d) accepting neither treatment. Above all, it is important to avoid being paternalistic and coercive by overelaborating the negative consequences of refusing an option that the staff feels is best. Respecting the patient's right to an informed autonomous choice in exercising some control over his or her destiny is crucial to achieving a dying process that allows the patient to meet an unavoidable end on his or her own terms.

That having been said, it bears repeating that not all segments of a pluralistic society place such value on self-determination (Working Group, 2000). Some patients will not want to make decisions about their end-of-life care, and will prefer to have the treatment staff use their own judgment about how to proceed. In such cases, it is up to the clinical staff to operate on a *best interest* principle and determine those treatments to provide or withhold that, on balance, will make the patient's passing least onerous.

It is important to remember that even for those who wish to have a hand in shaping how they will die, the choices are nonetheless rather circumscribed. This very circumstance, however, makes it all the more imperative that treatment providers make every effort to honor those choices the patient may have. As Rando (1984) pointed out, the individual is constantly forced to confront a loss of control throughout the dying process. He or she often feels powerless when in the grip of a progressive and debilitating illness. There may be no better way to combat this sense of powerlessness and loss of control than to do all that is feasible to allow the patient to make choices about his or her care.

The development of the doctrine of informed consent in the mid-20th century was a very important step forward in terms of introducing greater self-determination into health care decision making. It paved the way for patients to make decisions about shifting from curative to comfort care, which might prevent a more prolonged and agonizing death. It also provided the basis for advanced care planning in which one has the possibility, usually through a health care proxy or by doing an advance directive, to have one's values and choices respected at a time when one is no longer capable of making decisions. The rise of the hospice movement and of palliative care (for those who can access it) has also provided a welcome alternative to the technology-driven, cure-oriented, conventional medical system.

Too often, however, there is a reluctance on the part of an entrenched system to relinquish a curative approach with the terminally ill. If such an approach is relinquished, it often comes with an emotional withdrawal from the patient. Too often advance directives are not well executed or are ignored by a busy, paternalistically oriented system. In addition, mainstream medicine continues to withhold a more wholehearted embrace of hospice and palliative care for those at the end of life. Thus, many terminally ill patients have to struggle more than they should in order to obtain the type of care they prefer.

Although progress in the so-called *futility* debate seems to have been achieved (i.e., there is movement toward a fair process approach to resolving value conflicts), one still too frequently hears pronouncements of futility in an attempt to assert authority and end discussion. With regard to the rationing of scarce resources, we continue to know little about the selection process on the referral end. Nor do we know how reliably the recommended criteria for final selection are applied. We do know, however, that many in the United States do not have equal access to scarce resources or, for that matter, to life-sustaining treatment more generally because they are uninsured, underinsured, or belong to a less privileged or minority group.

As the Institute of Medicine's Committee on Care at the End of Life has noted, we live in an era of evidence-based practice (Field & Cassel, 1997). Public and private health insurers increasingly look to the results of clinical research for guidance on what types of care they will cover. Unfortunately, relatively little research has been done on end-of-life issues and care. The consequence of this situation is that each year hundreds of thousands of patients die in great discomfort and with very little choice about treatments that might ease their suffering.

Physical pain has been the only major symptom for which biomedical researchers and clinicians have collaborated on a large scale to develop pharmacologic interventions that can bring some relief. Other symptoms associated with dying, however, need not be considered an inevitable part of the process. Thus, hormonal agents may be able to alter the trajectory of anorexia, weight loss, and weakness, and thereby improve the patient's ability to function during the life that remains. Respiratory stimulants may be developed that could offer some relief for patients with dyspnea or shortness of breath. Further investigations into the interaction of cognitive and emotional symptoms with physical symptoms might lead to more timely and appropriate psychological and psychopharmacological interventions during the terminal phase of an illness (Field & Cassel, 1997). Developments in areas such as these could provide palliative care with more options and give patients a wider range of choices to alleviate the distress and misery associated with the dying process.

Although symptom relief is obviously of great significance to the dying patient, and we hope to see progress on this issue in future research, part of its importance may reside in the degree to which it allows the individual to have the remaining energy to maintain relationships with loved ones and to exercise some autonomous choice over the circumstances in which he or she dies. Dignity, for a great many people in our society, is linked to self-determination, taking responsibility for oneself, and keeping meaningful connections with those who matter for as long as possible. If dignity is to be wrested from the indignities of the dying process, then it is likely to be found in these personal and interpersonal experiences.

In this regard, Chochinov's (2001) proposal for a dignity-conserving model of palliative care (noted in chapter 1) has been a heartening development. His model calls for strategies and interventions that take into account individual differences in how a particular patient or family may perceive dignity and self-worth. It poses questions and offers possible interventions to assist the individual in conserving dignity through the preservation of his or her role in the family, through the determination of his or her legacy, through the maintenance of pride, through attention to concerns about the aftermath of one's death, and so forth. When psychologists and other members of the health care team foster such models of care, they indeed do a great service to the dying patient and his or her family.

Bouvia v. Superior Court, 179 Cal. App. 3d 1127, 225 Cal. Rptr. 297 (1986).

Brief of the American Medical Association et al., as *amici curia* in support of petitioners, at 6, *Washington v. Glucksberg*, 117 S. Ct. 2258 (1997) (No. 96–110).

Breitbart, W., Rosenfeld, B., & Passik, S. (1996). Interest in physician-assisted suicide among ambulatory HIV-infected patients. *American Journal of Psychiatry, 153,* 238–242.

Breitbart, W., Rosenfeld, B., Pessin, H., Kaim, M., Funesti-Esch, J., Galieta, M., et al. (2000). Depression, hopelessness, and desire for hastened death in terminally ill patients with cancer. *The Journal of the American Medical Association, 284,* 2907–2911.

Brody, H. (1992). Assisted death: A compassionate response to a medical failure. *The New England Journal of Medicine, 327,* 1384–1388.

Brown Medical School, Center for Gerontology and Health Care Research. (2000, October 1). *TIME: Toolkit of Instruments to Measure End-of-Life Care.* Retrieved November 17, 2002, from http://www.chcr.brown.edu/pcoc/toolkit.htm

Burke, F. (1996). Dying by the rules: Legal decisions at the end of life. *North Carolina Medical Journal, 57,* 386–389.

Burns, J., Mitchell, C., Griffith, J., & Truog, R. (2001). End-of-life care in the pediatric intensive care unit: Attitudes and practices of pediatric critical care physicians and nurses. *Critical Care Medicine, 29,* 658–664.

Burns, J., Mitchell, C., Outwater, K., Geller, M., Griffith, J., Todres, et al. (2000). End-of-life care in the pediatric intensive care unit after the forgoing of life-sustaining treatment. *Critical Care Medicine, 28,* 3060–3066.

Bursztajn, H., Harding, H., Jr., Gutheil, T., & Brodsky, A. (1991). Beyond cognition: The role of disordered affective states in impairing competence to consent to treatment. *Bulletin of the American Academy of Psychiatry and Law, 19,* 383–388.

Burt, R. (1997). The Supreme Court speaks: Not assisted suicide but a constitutional right to palliative care. *The New England Journal of Medicine, 337,* 1234–1236.

Butterfield-Picard, H., & Magno, J. (1982). Hospice the adjective, not the noun: The future of a national priority. *American Psychologist, 37,* 1254-1259.

Byock, I. (1996). The nature of suffering and the nature of opportunity at the end of life. *Clinics in Geriatric Medicine, 12,* 237–252.

Byock, I., & Merriman, M. (1998). Measuring quality of life for patients with terminal illness: The Missoula–VITAS quality of life index. *Palliative Medicine, 12,* 231–244.

California Probate Code, Section 4736 (West 2000).

Callahan, D. (1995). Frustrated mastery: The cultural context of death in America. *Western Journal of Medicine, 163,* 226–230.

Callahan, D. (1999a). Reasons, rationality, and ways of life. In J. Werth Jr. (Ed.), *Contemporary perspectives on rational suicide* (pp. 22–28). Philadelphia: Brunner/Mazel.

Callahan, J. (1999b). Rational suicide: Destructive to the common good. In J. Werth Jr. (Ed.), *Contemporary perspectives on rational suicide* (pp. 142–147). Philadelphia: Brunner/Mazel.

Canetto, S., & Hollenshead, J. (1999). Gender and physician-assisted suicide: An analysis of the Kevorkian cases, 1990–1997. *Omega, 40,* 165–208.

Capron, A. M. (1995, March–April). Baby Ryan and virtual futility. *Hastings Center Report, 25,* 20–21.

Caralis, P., Davis, B., Wright, K., & Marcial, W. (1993). The influence of ethnicity and race on attitudes toward advance directives, life-prolonging treatments, and euthanasia. *The Journal of Clinical Ethics, 4,* 155–165.

Carrese, J., & Rhodes, L. (1995). Western bioethics on the Navajo reservation. *Journal of the American Medical Association, 274,* 826–829.

Cassel, E. (1982). The nature of suffering and the goals of medicine. *The New England Journal of Medicine, 306,* 639–645.

Cassem, E. (1995). Depressive disorders in the medically ill: An overview. *Psychosomatics, 36,* S2–S10.

Centers for Disease Control and Prevention (1999). Mortality patterns: United States, 1997. *Journal of the American Medical Association, 282,* 1512–1513.

Chambers, C., Diamond, J., Perkel, R., & Lasch. L. (1994). Relationship of advance directives to hospital charges in a Medicare population. *Archives of Internal Medicine, 154,* 541–547.

Child Abuse Prevention and Treatment and Adoption Reform Act. Public Law, 98–457, (1984).

Chin, A., Hedberg, K., Higginson, G., & Fleming, D. (1999). Legalized physician-assisted suicide in Oregon: The first year's experience. *New England Journal of Medicine, 340,* 577–583.

Chochinov, H. (2000). Psychiatry and terminal illness. *Canadian Journal of Psychiatry, 45,* 143–150.

Chochinov, H. (2002). Dignity-conserving care: A new model for palliative care, helping the patient feel valued. *The Journal of the American Medical Association, 287,* 2253–2260.

Chochinov, H., Wilson, K., Enns, M., & Lander, S. (1998). *Psychosomatics, 39,* 366–370.

Christakis, N., & Iwashyna, T. (2000). Impact of individual and market factors on the timing of initiation of hospice terminal care. *Medical Care, 38,* 528–541.

Christakis, N., & Lamont, E. (2000). Extent and determinants of error in doctors' prognoses in terminally ill patients: Prospective cohort study. *British Medical Journal, 320,* 469–472.

Chynoweth, R., Tonge, J., & Armstrong, J. (1980). Suicide in Brisbane: A retrospective psychosocial study. *Australia and New Zealand Journal of Psychiatry, 14,* 37–45.

Clarke, O., Glasson, J., Epps, C., Jr., Plows, C., Ruff, V., August, A., et al. (1995). Ethical considerations in the allocation of organs and other scarce medical resources among patients. *Archives of Internal Medicine, 155,* 29–40.

Cohen, L., Steinberg, M., Hails, K., Dobscha, S., & Fischel, S. (2000). Psychiatric evaluation of death-hastening requests: Lessons from dialysis discontinuation. *Psychosomatics, 41,* 195–203.

Cohen, S. R., & Mount, B. (1992). Quality of life in terminal illness: Defining and measuring subjective well-being in the dying. *Journal of Palliative Care, 8,* 40–45.

Cohen, S. R., Mount, B., Bruera, E., Provost, M., Rowe, J., & Tong, K. (1997). Validity of the McGill Quality of Life Questionnaire in the palliative care setting: A multi-centre Canadian study demonstrating the importance of the existential domain. *Palliative Medicine, 11,* 3–20.

Cohen, S. R., Mount, B., Strobel, M., & Bui, F. (1995). The McGill Quality of Life Questionnaire: A measure of quality of life appropriate for people with advanced disease. A preliminary study of validity and acceptability. *Palliative Medicine, 9,* 207–219.

Cohen, S. R., Mount, B., Tomas, J., & Mount, L. (1996). Existential well-being is an important determinant of quality of life: Evidence from the McGill Quality of Life Questionnaire. *Cancer, 77,* 576–586.

Cole, M., & Bellevance, F. (1997). Depression in elderly medical patients: A meta-analysis of outcomes. *Canadian Medical Association Journal, 157,* 1055–1060.

Colt, G. (1991). *The enigma of suicide.* New York: Summit Books.

Commission on Aging with Dignity. (1998). *Five wishes.* Tallahassee, FL: Author.

Committee on Bioethics, American Academy of Pediatrics. (1994). Guidelines on forgoing life-sustaining treatment. *Pediatrics, 93,* 532–536.

Coombs Lee, B., & Werth, J., Jr. (2000). Observations on the first year of Oregon's Death with Dignity Act. *Psychology, Public Policy, and Law, 6,* 268–290.

Cotton, P. (1992). "Basic benefits" have many variations, tend to become political issues. *The Journal of the American Medical Association, 268,* 2139–2141.

Cournos, F. (1993). Do psychiatric patients need greater protection than medical patients when they consent to treatment? *Psychiatric Quarterly, 64,* 319–329.

Covinsky, K., Landefeld, S., Teno, J., Connors, A., Jr., Dawson, N., Youngner, S., et al. (1996). Is economic hardship on the families of the seriously ill associated with patient and surrogate care preferences? *Archives of Internal Medicine, 156,* 1737–1741.

Coyne, J., Fechner-Bates, S., & Schwenk, T. (1994). Prevalence, nature, and comorbidity of depressive disorders in primary care. *General Hospital Psychiatry, 16,* 267–276.

Crawley, L., Payne, R., Bolden, J., Payne, T., Washington, P., & Williams, S. (2000). Palliative and end-of-life care in the African American community. *Journal of the American Medical Association, 284,* 2518–2521.

Cruzan v. Director, Missouri Department of Health, 497 DS 261 (1990).

Daaleman, T., & VandeCreek, L. (2000). Placing religion and spirituality in end-of-life care. *The Journal of the American Medical Association, 284,* 2514–2517.

DeAngelis, T. (2002, March). More psychologists needed in end-of-life care. *Monitor on Psychology, 33,* 52–55.

Delmonico, F., Arnold, R., Scheper-Hughes, N., Siminoff, L., Kahn, J., & Youngner, S. (2002). Ethical incentives—not payment—for organ donation. *New England Journal of Medicine, 346,* 2002–2005.

Department of Veterans Affairs. (2000). *Pain as the 5th vital sign toolkit.* Washington, DC: Veterans Health Administration.

Drane, J. (1984). Competency to give an informed consent: A model for making clinical assessments. *Journal of the American Medical Association, 252,* 925–927.

Dresser, R., & Whitehouse, P. (1994). The incompetent patient on the slippery slope. *Hastings Center Report, 24,* 6–12.

Dunn, H. (1994). *Hard choices for loving people: CPR, artificial feeding, comfort measures only, and the patient with a life-threatening illness.* Herndon, VA: A & A Publishers.

Emanuel, E. (1996). Cost savings at the end of life: What do the data show? *Journal of the American Medical Association, 275,* 1907–1914.

Emanuel, E., & Emanuel, L. (1992). Proxy decision making for incompetent patients: An ethical and empirical analysis. *Journal of the American Medical Association, 267,* 2067–2071.

Emanuel, E., & Emanuel, L. (1994). The economics of dying: The illusion of cost savings at the end of life. *The New England Journal of Medicine, 330,* 540–544.

Emanuel, E., & Emanuel, L. (1998). The promise of a good death. *The Lancet, 351* (suppl. II), 21–29.

Emanuel, E., Fairclough, D., Daniels, E., & Claridge, B. (1996). Euthanasia and physician-assisted suicide: Attitudes and experiences of oncology patients, oncologists, and the public. *The Lancet, 347,* 1805–1810.

Emanuel, E., Fairclough, D., & Emanuel, L. (2000). Attitudes and desires related to euthanasia and physician-assisted suicide among terminally ill patients and their caregivers. *Journal of the American Medical Association, 284,* 2460–2468.

Emanuel, E., Fairclough, D., Slutsman, J., Alpert, H., Baldwin, D., & Emanuel, L. (1999). Assistance from family members, friends, paid caregivers, and volunteers in the care of terminally ill patients. *The New England Journal of Medicine, 341,* 956–963.

Emanuel, E., Fairclough, D., Slutsman, J., & Emanuel, L. (2000). Understanding economic and other burdens of terminal illness: The experience of patients and their caregivers. *Annals of Internal Medicine, 132,* 451–459.

Fagerlin, A., Ditto, P., Hawkins, N. A., Schneider, C., & Smucker, W. (2002). The use of advance directives in end-of-life decision making: Problems and possibilities. *American Behavioral Scientist, 46,* 268–283.

Farnsworth, M. (1990). Competency evaluations in a general hospital. *Psychosomatics, 31,* 60–66.

Farrenkopf, T., & Bryan, J. (1999). Psychological consultation under Oregon's 1994 Death with Dignity Act: Ethics and procedures. *Professional Psychology: Research and Practice, 30,* 245–249.

Ferrans, C., & Powers, M. (1985). Quality of life index: Development and psychometric properties. *Advanced Nursing Science, 8,* 15–24.

Field, M., & Cassel, C. (Eds.). (1997). *Approaching death: Improving care at the end of life.* Washington, DC: National Academy Press.

Fins, J. (1997). Advance directives and SUPPORT. *Journal of the American Geriatrics Society, 45,* 519–520.

Finucane, T., & Harper, M. (1996). Ethical decision-making near the end of life. *Clinics in Geriatric Medicine, 12,* 369–377.

Firshein, J. (1996). Oregon rationing experiment faces hard times. *Lancet, 347,* 1110.

Fohr, S. A. (1998). The double effect of pain medication: Separating myth from reality. *Journal of Palliative Medicine, 1,* 315–328.

Foley, K., & Hendin, H. (1999). The Oregon report: Don't ask, don't tell. *Hastings Center Report, 29,* 37–42.

Frankl, V. (1963). *Man's search for meaning.* New York: Washington Square Press.

Freeman, H., & Payne, R. (2000). Racial injustice in health care. *The New England Journal of Medicine, 342,* 1045–1047.

Fulbrook, P. (1994). Assessing mental competence of patients and relatives. *Journal of Advanced Nursing, 20,* 457–461.

Gamble, E., McDonald, P., & Lichstein, P. (1991). Knowledge, attitudes, and behavior of elderly persons regarding living wills. *Archives of Internal Medicine, 151,* 277–280.

Ganzini, L., Nelson, H., Schmidt, T., Kraemer, D., Delorit, M., & Lee, M. (2000). Physicians' experiences with the Oregon Death with Dignity Act. *The New England Journal of Medicine, 342,* 557–563.

Geiger, H. J. (1996). Race and health care: An American dilemma? *The New England Journal of Medicine, 335,* 815–816.

Gill, T., & Feinstein, A. (1994). A critical appraisal of the quality of quality-of-life measurements. *Journal of the American Medical Association, 272,* 619–626.

Gilson, A., & Joranson, D. (2002). U.S. policies relevant to the prescribing of opioid analgesics for the treatment of pain in patients with addictive disease. *The Clinical Journal of Pain, 18,* S91–S98.

Goldblum, P., & Martin, D. (1999). Principles for the discussion of life and death options with terminally ill clients with HIV. *Professional Psychology: Research and Practice, 30,* 187–197.

Gornick, M., Eggers, P., Reilly, T., Mentnech, R., Fitterman, L., Kucken, L., et al. (1996). Effects of race and income on mortality and use of services among Medicare beneficiaries. *The New England Journal of Medicine, 335,* 791–799.

Greer, D., & Mor, V. (1985). How Medicare is altering the hospice movement. *Hastings Center Report, 15* (October), 5–9.

Greer, D., & Mor, V. (1986). An overview of National Hospice Study findings. *Journal of Chronic Diseases, 39,* 5–7.

Greer, D., Mor, V., Morris, J., Sherwood, S., Kidder, D., & Birnbaum, H. (1986). An alternative in terminal care: Results of the National Hospice Study. *Journal of Chronic Diseases, 39,* 9–26.

Gregory, D. R. (1995). VA Network futility guidelines: A resource for decisions about withholding and withdrawing treatment. *Cambridge Quarterly of Healthcare Ethics, 4,* 546–548.

Grisso, T., & Appelbaum, P. (1992). *Manual for understanding treatment disclosures.* Worcester, MA: University of Massachusetts Medical School.

Grisso, T., & Appelbaum, P. (1993). *Manual for thinking rationally about treatment.* Worcester, MA: University of Massachusetts Medical School.

Grisso, T., & Appelbaum, P. (1995a). Comparison of standards for assessing patients' capacities to make treatment decisions. *American Journal of Psychiatry, 152,* 1033–1037.

Grisso, T., & Appelbaum, P. (1995b). The MacArthur Treatment Competence Study. III: Abilities of patients to consent to psychiatric and medical treatments. *Law and Human Behavior, 19,* 149–174.

Grisso, T., & Appelbaum, P. (1998). *Assessing competence to consent to treatment: A guide for physicians and other health professionals.* New York: Oxford University Press.

Grisso, T., Appelbaum, P., Mulvey, E., & Fletcher, K. (1995). The MacArthur Treatment Competence Study. II: Measures of abilities related to competence to consent to treatment. *Law and Human Behavior, 19,* 127–148.

Hafemeister, T., Keilitz, I., & Banks, S. (1991). The judicial role in life-sustaining medical treatment decisions. *Issues in Law and Medicine, 7,* 53–72.

Halevy, A., & Brody, B. (1996). A multi-institution collaborative policy on medical futility. *Journal of the American Medical Association, 276,* 571–574.

Haley, W., LaMonde, L., Han, B., Narramore, S., & Schonwetter, R. (2001). Family caregiving in hospice: Effects on psychological and health functioning among spousal caregivers of hospice patients with lung cancer or dementia. *Hospice Journal, 15,* 1–18.

Haley, W., Neimeyer, R., Larson, D., Kwilosz, D., & Kasl-Godley, J. (2003). *Clinical roles for psychologists in end-of-life care: Emerging models of practice.* Unpublished manuscript.

Hallenbeck, J., Goldstein, M. K., & Mebane, E. (1996). Cultural considerations of death and dying in the United States. *Clinics in Geriatric Medicine, 12,* 393–406.

Hammes, B., & Rooney, B. (1998). Death and end-of-life planning in one midwestern community. *Archives of Internal Medicine, 158,* 383–390.

Harris, J. (1998). *Clones, genes, and immortality.* New York: Oxford University Press.

Harris, J. (2000). Intimations of immortality. *Science, 288,* 59.

Hartman-Stein, P. (2001, July/August). Psychologists trying to overcome barriers to work with hospice patients. *The National Psychologist,* pp. 12–13.

Headley, J. (1991). The DNR decision. Part II: Ethical principles and application. *Issues in Nursing Practice, V,* 34–37.

Hedberg, K., Hopkins, D., & Southwick, K. (2002). Legalized physician-assisted suicide in Oregon, 2001. *The New England Journal of Medicine, 346,* 450–452.

Hendin, H. (1995). *Suicide in America.* New York: W. W. Norton and Company.

Hendin, H. (1999). Suicide, assisted suicide, and euthanasia. In D. Jacobs (Ed.), *The Harvard Medical School guide to suicide assessment and intervention.* (pp. 540–560). San Francisco, CA: Jossey-Bass.

Hern, H. E., Jr., Koenig, B., Moore, L. J., & Marshall, P. (1998). The difference that culture can make in end-of-life decision making. *Cambridge Quarterly of Healthcare Ethics, 7,* 27–40.

Higginson, I., & McCarthy, M. (1993). Validity of the support team assessment schedule: Do staff's ratings reflect those made by patients or their families? *Palliative Medicine, 7,* 219–228.

Hospice Foundation of America. (2002, February 20). *What is hospice?* Retrieved February 20, 2002, from http://www.hospicefoundation.org/what_is/

In the matter of Baby K, 16F3d 590 (4th Cir. 1994).

In re Quinlan, 755 A2A 647 (NJ), cert. denied, 429 U.S. 922 (1976).

Introcaso, D., & Lynn, J. (2002). Systems of care: Future reform. *Journal of Palliative Medicine, 5,* 255–257.

Jamison, S. (1996). When drugs fail: Assisted deaths and not-so-lethal drugs. *Journal of Pharmaceutical Care and Pain and Symptom Control, 4.* 223–243.

Jamison, S. (1997) *Assisted suicide: A decision-making guide for health professionals.* San Francisco: Jossey-Bass Publishers.

Jamison, S. (1999). Psychology and rational suicide: The special case of assisted dying. In J. Werth Jr. (Ed.), *Contemporary perspectives on rational suicide* (pp. 128–134). Philadelphia: Brunner/Mazel.

Janofsky, J., McCarthy, R., & Folstein, M. (1992). The Hopkins Competency Assessment Test: A brief method for evaluating patients' capacity to give informed consent. *Hospital and Community Psychiatry, 43,* 132–136.

Joranson, D., Gilson, A., Dahl, J., & Haddox, J. D. (2002). Pain management, controlled substances, and State Medical Board policy: A decade of change. *Journal of Pain and Symptom Management, 23,* 138–147.

Kahn, K., Pearson, M., Harrison, E., Desmond, K., Rogers, W., Rubenstein, L., et al. (1994). Health care for Black and poor hospitalized Medicare patients. *The Journal of the American Medical Association, 271,* 1169–1174.

Kamisar, Y. (1998). Physician-assisted suicide: The problems presented by the compelling, heart-wrenching case. *The Journal of Criminal Law and Criminology, 88,* 1121–1146.

Kane, R., Wales, J., Bernstein, L., Leibowitz, A., & Kaplan, S. (1984). A randomized controlled trial of hospice care. *Lancet, 1,* 890–894.

Kaplan, K., & Price, M. (1989). The clinician's role in competency evaluations. *General Hospital Psychiatry, 11,* 397–403.

Kaplan, K., Strang, J., & Ahmed, I. (1988). Dementia, mental retardation, and competency to make decisions. *General Hospital Psychiatry, 10,* 385–388.

Kaprio, J., Koskenvuo, M., & Rita, H. (1987). Mortality after bereavement: A prospective study of 95,647 widowed persons. *American Journal of Public Health, 77,* 283–287.

Karel, M. (2000). The assessment of values in medical decision making. *Journal of Aging Studies, 14,* 403–422.

Kelner, M. (1995). Activists and delegates: Elderly patients' preferences about control at the end of life. *Social Science and Medicine, 4,* 537–545.

Kleespies, P. (Ed.). (1998). *Emergencies in mental health practice: Evaluation and management.* New York: Guilford Press.

Kleespies, P., & Mori, D. (1998). Life and death decisions: Refusing life-sustaining treatment. In P. Kleespies (Ed.), *Emergencies in mental health practice: Evaluation and management* (pp. 145–173). New York: Guilford Press.

Kleespies, P., Hughes, D., & Gallacher, F. (2000). Suicide in the medically and terminally ill: Psychological and ethical considerations. *Journal of Clinical Psychology, 56,* 1153–1171.

Knaus, W., Wagner, D., Draper, E., Zimmerman, J., Bergner, M., Bastos, P., et al. (1991). The APACHE III prognostic system: Risk prediction of hospital mortality for critically ill hospitalized adults. *Chest, 100,* 1619–1636.

Koenig, H., & Blazer, D. (1992). Epidemiology of geriatric affective disorder. *Clinical Geriatric Medicine, 8,* 235–251.

Krakauer, E., Penson, R., Truog, R., King, L., Chabner, B., & Lynch, T. (2000). Sedation for intractable distress of a dying patient: Acute palliative care and the principle of double effect. *The Oncologist, 5,* 53–62.

Kutner, N. (1994). Is there bias in the allocation of treatment for renal failure? In H. McGee & C. Bradley (Eds.), *Quality of life following renal failure* (pp. 153–168). Langhorne, PA: Harwood.

Larson, D. (Ed.). (2001). *Finding our way: Living with dying in America.* Retrieved April 16, 2002, from http://www.findingourway.net

Lattanzi-Licht, M., & Connor, S. (1995). Care of the dying: The hospice approach. In H. Wass & R. Neimeyer (Eds.), *Dying: Facing the facts* (3rd ed., pp. 143–162). Washington, DC: Taylor and Francis.

Lavery, J., Boyle, J., Dickens, B., Maclean, H., & Singer, P. (2001). Origins of the desire for euthanasia and assisted suicide in people with HIV-1 or AIDS: A qualitative study. *The Lancet, 358,* 362–367.

Liao, Y., Mcgee, D., Cao, G., & Cooper, R. (2000). Quality of the last year of life of older adults: 1986 vs. 1993. *Journal of the American Medical Association, 283,* 512–518.

Luce, J., & Alpers, A. (2001). End-of-life care: What do the American courts say? *Critical Care Medicine, 29*(2, Suppl.), N40–N45.

Lynn, J. (2001). Serving patients who may die soon and their families: The role of hospice and other services. *The Journal of the American Medical Association, 285,* 925–932.

Lynn, J., Nolan, K., Kabcenell, A., Weissman, D., Milne, C., & Berwick, D. (2002). Reforming care for persons near the end of life: The promise of quality improvement. *Annals of Internal Medicine, 137,* 117–122.

Lynn, J., O'Connor, M. A., Dulac, J., Roach, M. J., Ross, C., & Wasson, J. (1999). Medicaring: Development and test marketing of a supportive care benefit for older people. *The Journal of the American Geriatrics Society, 47,* 1058–1064.

Lynn, J., Teno, J., Phillips, R., Wu, A., Desbiens, N., Harrold, J., et al. (1997).

Perceptions by family members of the dying experience of older and seriously ill patients. *Annals of Internal Medicine, 126,* 97–106.

Maddi, S. (1990). Prolonging life by heroic measures: A humanistic existential perspective. In P. T. Costa Jr., & G. R. VandenBos (Eds.), *Psychological aspects of serious illness: Chronic conditions, fatal diseases, and clinical care* (pp. 155–184). Washington, DC: American Psychological Association.

Maddox, P. (1998, December 31). Administrative ethics and the allocation of scarce resources. *Online Journal of Issues in Nursing.* Retrieved January 20, 2002, from http://www.nursingworld.org/ojin/topic8/topic8_5.htm

Marson, D., Ingram, K., Cody, H., & Harrell, L. (1995). Assessing the competency of patients with Alzheimer's disease under different legal standards: A prototype instrument. *Archives of Neurology, 52,* 949–954.

Marson, D., Schmitt, F., Ingram, K., & Harrell, L. (1994). Determining the competency of Alzheimer patients to consent to treatment and research. *Alzheimer Disease and Associated Disorders, 8,* 5–18.

Martin, D., Thiel, E., & Singer, P. (2002). A new model of advance care planning: Observations from people with HIV. *Archives of Internal Medicine,* in press.

Marwit, S. (1997). Professional psychology's role in hospice care. *Professional Psychology: Research and Practice, 28,* 457–463.

Mayo, D. (1992). What is being predicted? The definition of "suicide." In R. Maris, A. Berman, J. Maltsberger, & R. Yufit (Eds.), *Assessment and prediction of suicide* (pp. 88–101). New York: Guilford Press.

McCamish, M., & Crocker, N. (1993). Enteral and parenteral nutrition support of terminally ill patients: Practical and ethical perspectives. *The Hospice Journal, 9,* 107–129.

McCracken, L., & Turk, D. (2002). Behavioral and cognitive–behavioral treatment for chronic pain: Outcome, predictors of outcome, and treatment process. *Spine, 27,* 2564–2573.

McCrary, S., & Walman, A. (1990). Procedural paternalism in competency determination. *Law, Medicine, and Health Care, 18,* 108–113.

McKnight, D., & Bellis, M. (1992). Forgoing life-sustaining treatment for adult, developmentally disabled, public wards: A proposed statute. *American Journal of Law and Medicine, 18*(3), 203–232.

Meier, D., Emmons, C., Wallenstein, S., Quill, T., Morrison, R. S., & Cassel, C. (1998). A national survey of physician-assisted suicide and euthanasia in the United States. *The New England Journal of Medicine, 338,* 1193–1201.

Meisel, A., Jernigan, J., & Youngner, S. (1999). Prosecutors and end-of-life decision making. *Archives of Internal Medicine, 159,* 1089–1095.

Melzer, D., McWilliams, B., Brayne, C., Johnson, T., & Bond, J. (2000). Socioeconomic status and the expectation of disability in old age: Estimates for England. *Journal of Epidemiology and Community Health, 54,* 286–292.

Miles, S. (1991). Informed demand for "nonbeneficial" medical treatment. *The New England Journal of Medicine, 325,* 512–515.

Miller, F., & Meier, D. (1998). Voluntary death: A comparison of terminal dehydration and physician-assisted suicide. *Annals of Internal Medicine, 128,* 559–562.

Mishara, B. (1999). Synthesis of research and evidence on factors affecting the desire of terminally ill or seriously chronically ill persons to hasten death. *Omega, 39,* 1–70.

Mishkin, B. (1989). Determining the capacity for making health care decisions. In B. Billig & P. Rabins (Eds.), *Issues in geriatric psychiatry: Advances in psychosomatic medicine* (Vol. 19, pp. 151–166). Basil, Switzerland: Karger.

Molloy, W., Guyatt, G., Russo, R., Goeree, R., O'Brien, B., Bedard, M., et al. (2000). Systematic implementation of an advance directive program in nursing homes. *Journal of the American Medical Association, 283,* 1437–1444.

Mor, V., & Kidder, D. (1985). Cost savings in hospice: Final results of the National Hospice Study. *Health Services Research, 20,* 407–422.

Morris, J., Mor, V., Goldberg, R., Sherwood, S., Greer, D., & Hiris, J. (1986). The effect of treatment setting and patient characteristics on pain in terminal cancer patients: A report from the National Hospice Study. *Journal of Chronic Diseases, 39,* 27–35.

Morrison, R. S., Wallenstein, S., Natale, D., Senzel, R., & Huang, L. (2000). "We don't carry that:" Failure of pharmacies in predominantly nonwhite neighborhoods to stock opioid analgesics. *The New England Journal of Medicine, 342,* 1023–1026.

Moye, J. (2000). Mr. Franks refuses surgery: Cognition and values in competency determination in complex cases. *Journal of Aging Studies, 14,* 385–401.

Natanson v. Kline, 350 P.2d 1093 (1960).

National Center for Ethics, Veterans Health Administration. (2000, December). *Do-Not-Resuscitate orders and medical futility: A report of the National Ethics Committee of the Veterans Health Administration.* Washington, DC: Veterans Health Administration, Department of Veterans Affairs.

National Center for Health Statistics. (2000, July 24). Gun deaths among children and teens drop sharply. *HHS News.* Washington, DC: U.S. Department of Health and Human Services News Release.

National Hospice Organization (NHO). (1995). *An analysis of the cost savings of the Medicare Hospice Benefit.* NHO Item Code 712901. Miami, FL: Lewin-VHI.

Navarro, V. (1990). Race or class versus race and class: Mortality differentials in the United States. *The Lancet, 336,* 1238–1240.

Nicholson, B., & Matross, G. (1989, May). Facing reduced decision-making capacity in health care: Methods for maintaining client self-determination. *Social Work,* pp. 234–238.

Niemeyer, R. (Ed.). (2001). *Meaning reconstruction and the experience of loss.* Washington, DC: American Psychological Association.

Niemeyer, R., & Van Brunt, D. (1995). Death anxiety. In H. Wass & R. Niemeyer (Eds.), *Dying: Facing the facts* (pp. 49–88). Washington, DC: Taylor and Francis.

Normand, C. (1994). Health care resource allocation and the management of renal failure. In H. McGee & C. Bradley (Eds.), *Quality of life following renal failure* (pp. 145–152). Langhorne, PA: Harwood.

Nuland, S. (1993). *How we die: Reflections on life's final chapter*. New York: Vintage Books.

Ogden, R. (2001). Nonphysician assisted suicide: The technological imperative of the deathing counterculture. *Death Studies, 25*, 387–401.

Olbrisch, M. (1996). Picking winners and grooming the dark horse: Psychologists evaluate and treat organ transplant patients. *The Health Psychologist, 18*, 10–11.

Oregon Death with Dignity Act. (1995). *Oregon Revised Statute* 127.800–127.995.

Orentlicher, D. (1997). The Supreme Court and physician-assisted suicide: Rejecting assisted suicide but embracing euthanasia. *The New England Journal of Medicine, 337*, 1236–1239.

Orentlicher, D. (2000). The implementation of Oregon's Death with Dignity Act: Reassuring, but more data are needed. *Psychology, Public Policy, and Law, 6*, 489–502.

Parry, J. (1990). The court's role in decision making involving incompetent refusals of life-sustaining care and psychiatric medications. *Mental and Physical Disability Law Reporter, 14*, 468–476.

The Patient Self-Determination Act (OBRA 1990). (1990). Public Law 101-508, Sect 4206, 4751 (OBRA), 42 USC 1395 cc(a) et seq.

Pearlman, R., Starks, H., Cain, K., Cole, W., Rosengren, D., & Patrick, D. (2001). *Your life, your choices: Planning for future medical decisions: How to prepare a personalized living will*. Retrieved December 10, 2001, from http://www.va.gov/resdev/programs/hsrd/ylyc.htm

Peruzzi, N., Canapary, A., & Bongar, B. (1996). Physician-assisted suicide: The role of mental health professionals. *Ethics and Behavior, 6*, 353–366.

Peterson, E., Wright, S., Daley, J., & Thibault, G. (1994). Racial variation in cardiac procedure use and survival following acute myocardial infarction in the Department of Veterans Affairs. *The Journal of the American Medical Association, 271*, 1175–1180.

Plows, C., Tenery, R., Jr., Hartford, A., Miller, D., Morse, L., Rakatansky, H., et al. (1999). Medical futility in end-of-life care: Report of the Council on Ethical and Judicial Affairs. *Journal of the American Medical Association, 281*, 937–941.

Powell, J., & Cohen, A. (1994). The right to die. *Issues in law and medicine, 10*, 169–182.

Prendergast, T. (1995). Futility and the common cold: How requests for antibiotics can illuminate care at the end of life. *Chest, 107*, 836–844.

Prendergast, T. (2001). Advance care planning: Pitfalls, progress, promise. *Critical Care Medicine, 29(Suppl. 2)*, N34–N39.

The President's Commission for the Study of Ethical Problems in Medicine and Biomedical and Behavioral Research. (1983). *Deciding to forego life-sustaining treatment: Ethical, medical, and legal issues in treatment decisions*. PB-83236836. Springfield, VA: The National Technical Information Service.

Prigerson, H., Bierhals, A., Kasl, S., Reynolds, C., III, Shear, M. K., Day, N., et al. Traumatic grief as a risk factor for mental and physical morbidity. *American Journal of Psychiatry, 154*, 616–623.

Printz, L. (1992). Terminal dehydration: A compassionate treatment. *Archives of Internal Medicine, 152*, 697–700.

Quill, T. (1989). Utilization of nasogastric feeding tubes in a group of chronically ill, elderly patients in a community hospital. *Archives of Internal Medicine, 149*, 1937–1941.

Quill, T. (1991). Death and dignity: A case of individualized decision making. *The New England Journal of Medicine, 324*, 691–694.

Quill, T. (1993). The ambiguity of clinical intentions. *The New England Journal of Medicine, 329*, 1039–1040.

Quill, T., & Byock, I. (2000). Responding to intractable terminal suffering: The role of terminal sedation and voluntary refusal of food and fluids. *Annals of Internal Medicine, 132*, 408–414.

Quill, T., Cassel, C., & Meier, D. (1992). Care of the hopelessly ill: Proposed clinical criteria for physician-assisted suicide. *The New England Journal of Medicine, 327*, 1380–1384.

Quill, T., Dresser, R., & Brock, D. (1997). The rule of double effect: A critique of its role in end-of-life decision making. *The New England Journal of Medicine, 337*, 1768–1771.

Quill, T., Lo, B., & Brock, D. (1997). Palliative options of last resort: A comparison of voluntarily stopping eating and drinking, terminal sedation, physician-assisted suicide, and voluntary active euthanasia. *The Journal of the American Medical Association, 278*, 2099–2104.

Rando, T. (1984). *Grief, dying, and death: Clinical interventions for caregivers.* Champaign, IL: Research Press.

Rando, T. (1986). *Loss and anticipatory grief.* Lexington, MA: Lexington Books.

Rando, T. (1995). Grief and mourning: Accommodating to loss. In H. Wass & R. Niemeyer (Eds.), *Dying: Facing the facts* (pp. 211–241). Washington, DC: Taylor and Francis.

Rando, T. (Ed.). (2000). *Clinical dimensions of anticipatory mourning: Theory and practice in working with the dying, their loved ones, and their caregivers.* Champaign, IL: Research Press.

Rich, C., Young, D., & Fowler, R. (1986). San Diego suicide study. I: Young vs. old subjects. *Archives of General Psychiatry, 43*, 577–582.

Rihmer, Z., Rutz, W., & Pihlgren, H. (1995). Depression and suicide in Gotland: An intensive study of all suicides before and after a depression-training programme for general practitioners. *Journal of Affective Disorders, 35*, 147–152.

Roff, S., & Moore, C. (2001, December 10). Advanced illness coordinated care: A model for social work intervention. *Social Work Today*, pp. 10–12.

Roscoe, L., Malphurs, J., Dragovic, L., & Cohen, D. (2001). A comparison of characteristics of Kevorkian euthanasia cases and physician-assisted suicides in Oregon. *The Gerontologist, 41*, 439–446.

Rosenfeld, B. (2000). Methodological issues in assisted suicide and euthanasia research. *Psychology, Public Policy, and Law, 6*, 559–574.

Roth, L., Meisel, A., & Lidz, C. (1977). Tests of competency to consent to treatment. *American Journal of Psychiatry, 134*, 279–284.

Rutz, W., von Knorring, L., & Walinder, J. (1989). Frequency of suicide on Gotland after systematic postgraduate education of general practitioners. *Acta Psychiatrica Scandinavica, 80*, 151–154.

Rutz, W., von Knorring, L., & Walinder, J. (1992). Long-term effects of an educational program for general practitioners given by the Swedish Committee for the Prevention and Treatment of Depression. *Acta Psychiatrica Scandinavica, 58*, 83–88.

Schade, C., Jones, E., & Wittlin, B. (1998). A 10-year review of the validity and clinical utility of depression screening. *Psychiatric Services, 49*, 55–60.

Schmidt, V. (1998). Selection of recipients for donor organs in transplant medicine. *Journal of Medicine and Philosophy, 23*, 50–74.

Schneiderman, L. (1993). Futility in practice. *Archives of Internal Medicine, 153*, 437–441.

Schneiderman, L., Kronick, R., Kaplan, R., Anderson, J., & Langer, R. (1992). Effects of offering advance directives on medical treatments and costs. *Annals of Internal Medicine, 117*, 599–606.

Schulman, K., Berlin, J., Harless, W., Kerner, J., Sistrunk, S., Gersh, B., et al. (1999). The effect of race and sex on physicians' recommendations for cardiac catheterization. *The New England Journal of Medicine, 340*, 618–626.

Schwenzer, K., Smith, W., & Durbin, C. (1993). Selective application of cardiopulmonary resuscitation improves survival rates. *Anesthesiology Analog, 76*, 478–484.

Seale, C. (2000). Changing patterns of death and dying. *Social Science & Medicine, 51*, 917–930.

Searight, H. (1992). Assessing patient competence for medical decision making. *American Family Physician, 45*, 751–759.

Seckler, A., Meier, D., Mulvihill, M., & Paris, B. (1991). Substituted judgment: How accurate are proxy prediction? *Annals of Internal Medicine, 115*, 92–98.

Sehgal, A., Galbraith, A., Chesney, M., Schoenfeld, P., Charles, G., & Lo, B. (1992). How strictly do dialysis patients want their advance directives followed? *Journal of the American Medical Association, 267*, 59–63.

Sigman, G., & O'Connor, C. (1991). Exploration for physicians of the mature minor doctrine. *The Journal of Pediatrics, 119*, 520–525.

Simon, E., & Folen, R. (2001). The role of the psychologist on the multidisciplinary pain management team. *Professional Psychology: Research and Practice, 32*, 125–134.

Simon, R. (1994). The law and psychiatry. In R. Hales, S. Yudofsky, & J. Talbott (Eds.), *The American Psychiatric Press textbook of psychiatry* (2nd ed., pp. 1297–1335). Washington, DC: American Psychiatric Press.

Singer, P. (1992). Nephrologists' experience with and attitudes toward decisions to forego dialysis. *Journal of the American Society of Nephrology, 7*, 1235–1240.

Singer, P., Martin, D., & Kelner, M. (1999). Quality end-of-life care: Patients' perspectives. *Journal of the American Medical Association, 281*, 163–168.

Singer, P., Martin, D., Lavery, J., Thiel, E., Kelner, M., & Mendelssohn, D. (1998). Reconceptualizing advance care planning from the patient's perspective. *Archives of Internal Medicine, 158*, 879–884.

Slome, L., Mitchell, T., Charlebois, E., Benevedes, J., & Abrams, D. (1997). Physician-assisted suicide and patients with human immunodeficiency virus disease. *The New England Journal of Medicine, 336*, 417–421.

Snyder, J., & Swartz, M. (1993). Deciding to terminate treatment: A practical guide for physicians. *Journal of Critical Care, 8*, 177–185.

Stanley, B. (1983). Senile dementia and informed consent. *Behavioral Sciences and the Law, 1*, 57–71.

The Study to Understand Prognoses and Preferences for Outcomes and Risks of Treatment (SUPPORT) Principal Investigators. (1995). A controlled trial to improve care for seriously ill hospitalized patients: The Study to Understand Prognoses and Preferences for Outcomes and Risks of Treatments (SUPPORT). *Journal of the American Medical Association, 274*, 1591–1598.

Sullivan, A., Hedberg, K., & Fleming, D. (2000). Legalized physician-assisted suicide in Oregon: The second year. *The New England Journal of Medicine, 342*, 598–604.

Sullivan, A., Hedberg, K., & Hopkins, D. (2001). Legalized physician-assisted suicide in Oregon, 1998–2000. *The New England Journal of Medicine, 344*, 605–607.

Sullivan, M., & Youngner, S. (1994). Depression, competence, and the right to refuse lifesaving medical treatment. *American Journal of Psychiatry, 151*, 971–978.

Sulmasy, D., Terry, P., Weisman, C., Miller, D., Stallings, R., Vettese, M., et al. (1998). The accuracy of substituted judgments in patients with terminal diagnoses. *Annals of Internal Medicine, 128*, 621–629.

Tan, S. Y. (1995). Medical decisions at the end-of-life: Lessons from America. *Hawaii Medical Journal, 54*, 514–520.

Tax Equity and Fiscal Responsibility Act. Public Law No. 97-248. (1982).

Teno, J., Licks, S., Lynn, J., Wenger, N., Connors, A., Jr., Phillips, R., et al. (1997). Do advance directives provide instructions that direct care? *Journal of the American Geriatric Society, 45*, 508–512.

Teno, J., Lynn, J., Connors, A., Wenger, N., Phillips, R., Alzola, C., et al. (1997). The illusion of end-of-life resource savings with advance directives. *Journal of the American Geriatrics Society, 45*, 513–518.

Teno, J., Lynn, J., Wenger, N., Phillips, R., Murphy, D., Connors, A., Jr., et al. (1997). Advance directives for seriously ill hospitalized patients: Effectiveness with the Patient Self-Determination Act and the SUPPORT intervention. *Journal of the American Geriatrics Society, 45*, 500–507.

Terkel, S. (2001). *Will the circle be unbroken? Reflections on death, rebirth, and hunger for faith.* New York: The New Press.

Texas Health & Safety Code, Section 166 (1999).

Thibault, G. (1997). Prognosis and clinical predictive models for critically ill patients. In M. Field & C. Cassell (Eds.), *Approaching death: Improving care at the end of life* (pp. 358–362). Washington, DC: National Academy Press.

Tobin, D. (with Lindsey, K.) (1999). *Peaceful dying: The step-by-step guide to preserving your dignity, your choice, and your inner peace at the end of life.* Reading, MA: Perseus Books.

Tobin, D., & Larson, D. (2000). *Advanced illness coordinated care program: Training manual.* Altamont, NY: The Life Institute Press.

Tonelli, M. (1996). Pulling the plug on living wills: A critical analysis of advance directives. *Chest, 110,* 816–822.

Tresch, D., Heudebert, G., Kutty, K., Ohlert, J., Van Beek, K., & Masi, A. (1994). Cardiopulmonary resuscitation in elderly patients hospitalized in the 1990s: A favorable outcome. *Journal of the American Geriatrics Society, 42,* 137–141.

Tresch, D., Neahring, J., Duthie, E., Mark, D., Kartes, S., & Aufderheide, T. (1993). Outcomes of cardiopulmonary resuscitation in nursing homes: Can we predict who will benefit? *The American Journal of Medicine, 95,* 123–130.

Truog, R. (1995). Progress in the futility debate. *The Journal of Clinical Ethics, 6,* 128–132.

Truog, R. (2000). Futility in pediatrics: From case to policy. *The Journal of Clinical Ethics, 11,* 136–141.

Truog, R., Berde, C., Mitchell, C., & Grier, H. (1992). Barbiturates in the care of the terminally ill. *The New England Journal of Medicine, 327,* 1678–1682.

Truog, R., Brett, A., & Frader, J. (1992). The problem with futility. *The New England Journal of Medicine, 326,* 1560–1564.

Tulsky, J., Fischer, G., Rose, M., & Arnold, R. (1998). Opening the black box: How do physicians communicate about advance directives? *Annals of Internal Medicine, 129,* 441–449.

Turk, D., & Okifuji, A. (2002). Psychological factors in chronic pain: Evolution and revolution. *Journal of Consulting and Clinical Psychology, 70,* 678–690.

United Network of Organ Sharing (2001, March). National organ transplant waiting list tops 75,000. Retrieved January 21, 2002, from UNOS News Release at http://www.unos.org/Newsroom/archive_newsrelease_20010309_75000.htm

Vacco v. Quill, 521 U.S. 793 (1997).

VandenBos, G., DeLeon, P., & Pallak, M. (1982). An alternative to traditional medical care for the terminally ill: Humanitarian, policy, and political issues in hospice care. *American Psychologist, 37,* 1245–1248.

van der Maas, P., van Delden, J., Pijnenborg, L., & Looman, C. (1991). Euthanasia and other medical decisions concerning the end of life. *The Lancet, 338,* 669–674.

van der Maas, P., van der Wal, G., Haverkate, I., de Graff, C., Kester, J., Onwuteaka-Philipsen, B., et al. (1996). Euthanasia, physician-assisted suicide, and other medical practices involving the end of life in the Netherlands, 1990–1995. *The New England Journal of Medicine, 335,* 1699–1705.

van der Wal, G., van der Maas, P., Bosma, J., Onwuteaka-Philipsen, B., Willems, D., Haverkate, I., et al. (1996). Evaluation of the notification procedure for physician-assisted death in the Netherlands. *The New England Journal of Medicine, 335,* 1706–1711.

Venesy, B. (1994). A clinician's guide to decision-making capacity and ethically sound medical decisions. *American Journal of Physical Medicine and Rehabilitation, 73,* 219–226.

Veterans Affairs National Headquarters Bioethics Committee. (1996, May). *Ethics advisory committees* (VA National Headquarters Bioethics Committee Report). White River Junction, VT: VA National Center for Clinical Ethics.

Wachter, R., & Lo, B. (1993). Advanced directives for patients with human immunodeficiency virus infection. *Critical Care Clinics, 9,* 125–136.

Walker, A., & Charlton, K. (1999). Evaluating changes in life expectancy and survival in the elderly. *Journal of Evaluation in Clinical Practice, 5,* 57–63.

Wallston, K., Burger, C., Smith, R. A., & Baugher, R. (1988). Comparing the quality of death for hospice and nonhospice cancer patients. *Medical Care, 26,* 177–182.

Washington v. Glucksberg, 521 U.S. 702 (1997).

Watson, R. (2002). First Belgian to use new euthanasia law provokes storm of protest. *British Medical Journal, 325,* 854.

Weber, W. (2001). Netherlands legalize euthanasia. *The Lancet, 357,* 1189.

Weeks, W., Kofoed, L., Wallace, A., & Welch. H. G. (1994). Advance directives and the cost of terminal hospitalization. *Archives of Internal Medicine, 154,* 2077–2083.

Wells, K., Golding, J., & Burnam, A. (1988). Psychiatric disorder in a sample of the general population with or without chronic medical conditions. *American Journal of Psychiatry, 145,* 976–981.

Wehrwein, P. (Ed.). (1999). Aging: Great expectations. *Harvard Health Letter, 25,* 1–2.

Weithorn, L., & Campbell, S. (1982). The competency of children and adolescents to make informed treatment decisions. *Child Development, 53,* 1589–1598.

Werth, J., Jr. (1999a). Introduction to the issue of rational suicide. In J. Werth Jr. (Ed.), *Contemporary perspectives on rational suicide* (pp. 1–9). Philadelphia: Brunner/Mazel.

Werth, J., Jr. (1999b). Mental health professionals and assisted death: Perceived ethical obligations and proposed guidelines for practice. *Ethics and Behavior, 9,* 159–183.

Werth, J., Jr. (2000). How do the mental health issues differ in the withholding/withdrawing of treatment versus assisted death? *Omega, 41,* 259–278.

Werth, J., Jr. (2002). Reinterpreting the Controlled Substances Act: Predictions for the effect on pain relief. *Behavioral Sciences and the Law, 20,* 287–305.

Werth, J., Jr., Benjamin, G. A., & Farrenkopf, T. (2000). Request for physician-assisted death: Guidelines for assessing mental capacity and impaired judgment. *Psychology, Public Policy, & Law, 6,* 348–372.

Werth, J., Jr., & Blevins, D. (2002). Public policy and end-of-life care. *American Behavioral Scientist, 46,* 401–417.

Werth, J., Jr., Blevins, D., Toussaint, K., & Durham, M. (2002). The influence of cultural diversity in end-of-life care and decisions. *American Behavioral Scientist, 46,* 204–219.

Werth, J., Jr. & Cobia, D. (1995). Empirically based criteria for rational suicide: A survey of psychotherapists. *Suicide and Life-Threatening Behavior, 25,* 231–240.

Werth, J., Jr. & Liddle, B. (1994). Psychotherapists' attitudes toward suicide. *Psychotherapy: Theory, Research, and Practice, 31,* 440–448.

Wilson, W., Smedira, N., Fink, C., McDowell, J., & Luce, J. (1992). Ordering and administering of sedatives and analgesics during the withholding and withdrawal of life support from critically ill patients. *The Journal of the American Medical Association, 267,* 949–953.

Wolf, S., Boyle, P., Callahan, D., Fins, J., Jennings, B., Nelson, J., et al. (1991). Special report: Sources of concern about the patient self-determination act. *New England Journal of Medicine, 325,* 1666–1671.

Worden, J. W. (1991). *Grief counseling and grief therapy: A handbook for the mental health practitioner.* New York: Springer Publishing Company.

Wyden, R. (2000). Steps to improve quality of life for people who are dying. *Psychology, Public Policy, and Law, 6,* 575–581.

Zawacki, B. (1995). The "futility debate" and the management of Gordian knots. *The Journal of Clinical Ethics, 6,* 112–127.

Zerzan, J., Stearns, S., & Hanson, L. (2000). Access to palliative care and hospice in nursing homes. *Journal of the American Medical Association, 284,* 2489–2494.

AUTHOR INDEX

Abrams, D., 95
Ahmed, I., 52
Allumbaugh, D. L., 159
Alpers, A., 35, 36–37
American Academy of Pediatrics, 51
American Geriatric Society, 14, 16
American Medical Assoication (AMA), 106
American Psychological Assoication Working
 Group on Assisted Suicide, 4
American Society for Bioethics and
 Humanities, 160
Anderson, J., 22
Angell, M., 96, 98
Annas, G., 64, 161
APA Working Group, 20, 62, 86, 162, 165
Appelbaum, P., 34, 37–44, 47, 48, 49–50, 59,
 85, 155
Armstrong, J., 83
Arnold, R., 74–75, 118, 149
Asch, D., 53, 62
Auerbach, V., 40, 41
Awoke, S., 67
Ayanian, J., 126, 127

Back, A., 81, 84, 88, 94–95, 106
Baer, W., 139
Banja, J., 40, 41
Banks, S., 57
Battin, M., 18, 19, 21, 27–32, 63, 83, 85, 86,
 89, 91, 102, 103, 165
Baugher, R. 134–135
Bean, G., 47, 48
Beauchamp, T., 28–34, 69, 71, 78, 90, 91,
 94, 98–101, 107, 111, 112, 117, 119,
 121, 123, 124
Bellevance, F., 150
Bellis, M., 52, 57
Benevedes, J., 95
Benjamin, G. A., 46, 100, 154
Benoliel, J. Q., 138
Bentivegna, S., 47
Berde, C., 65, 113
Bernstein, L., 22
Black, D., 14
Blazer, D., 150
Blevins, D., 6, 28, 138, 139, 143

Block, S., 85, 86, 89, 150, 164
Boisaubin, E., 57–58
Bond, J., 11
Bongar, B., 150
Boyle, J., 87, 88, 89, 148
Brayne, C., 11
Breitbart, W., 3, 87, 153
Brett, A., 111–112
Brock, D., 63, 65, 66
Brodsky, A., 46
Brody, B., 115
Brody, H., 82, 88, 102
Bryan, J., 61
Bui, F., 15
Burger, C., 134–135
Burke, F., 35
Burnam, A., 150
Burns, J., 46, 57, 64
Bursztajn, H., 46
Burt, R., 37
Butterfield-Picard, H., 4, 129, 133
Byock, I., 15, 25, 26, 64, 65, 106, 163, 164

Callahan, D., 24, 82–85, 109
Callahan, J., 83
Campbell, S., 51
Canapary, A., 150
Canetto, S., 91–93
Cao, G., 14
Capron, A. M., 112
Caralis, P., 20, 142
Carrese, J., 21,
Cassel, C., 4, 16, 22, 23–24, 55, 58–59, 99–101,
 110, 123, 125, 130, 131, 137, 139, 140,
 141, 142, 152, 166, 167
Cassel, L., 163, 164
Cassem, E., 85, 150
Center for Gerontology and Health Care
 Research, 15
Centers for Disease Control, 11, 128
Chambers, C., 22
Charlebois, E., 95
Charlton, K., 11
Childress, J., 28–34, 69, 71, 78, 90, 91, 94,
 98–101, 107, 111, 112, 117, 119, 121,
 123, 124

Gutheil, T., 46

Haddox, J. D., 132
Hafemeister, T., 57
Hails, K., 61
Halevy, A., 115
Haley, W., 6, 135, 141, 148, 149–150, 151, 154
Hallenbeck, J., 6, 20, 21
Hammes, B., 75, 76, 149
Han, B.,141
Hansen-Flaschen, J., 53, 62
Hanson, L., 17, 138–140
Harding, H., 46
Harper, M., 55, 114
Harrell, L., 48
Harris, J., 12, 13
Hartman-Stein, P., 152
Hawkins, N. A., 71
Headley, J., 32
Hedberg, K., 88, 95
Hendin, H., 86, 96, 97, 101
Hern, H. E., 6
Higginson, G., 95
Higginson, I., 26
Hollenshead, J., 91–93
Hopkins, D., 88, 95
Hospice Foundation of America, 130
Hoyt, W., 159
Huang, L., 132
Hughes, D., 63, 78, 82, 84

Ingram, K., 48
Introcaso, D., 131
Iwashyna, T., 142

Jamison, S., 83, 90, 96, 101
Janofsky, J., 47, 48
Jernigan, J., 99
Johnson, T., 11
Jolley, D., 14
Jones, E., 150
Joranson, D., 132

Kahn, K., 126
Kamisar, Y., 99
Kane, R., 22
Kaplan, K., 47, 52
Kaplan, R., 22

Kaplan, S., 22
Kaprio, J., 158
Karel, M., 45, 46
Kasl-Godley, J., 6, 135, 148, 149–150, 151, 154
Keilitz, I., 57
Kelner, M., 16, 17
Kidder, D., 22
Kleespies, P., 18–19, 41, 43, 49, 63, 78, 82, 84, 86
Knaus, W., 59
Koenig, B., 6
Koenig, H., 150
Kofoed, L., 22
Koskenvuo, M., 158
Krakauer, E., 65
Kronick, R., 22
Kwilosz, D., 6, 135, 148, 149–150, 151, 154

LaMonde, L., 141
Lamont, E., 58, 139
Lander, S., 153
Langer, R., 22
Lanken, P., 53, 62
Larson, D., 6, 135, 144, 145, 148–151, 154
Lasch, L., 22
Lattanzi-Licht, M., 131, 135–136
Lavery, J., 87, 88, 89, 148
Lebowitz, A., 22
Liao, Y., 14
Lichstein, P., 72–73
Licks, S., 70, 72
Liddle, B., 84
Lidz, C., 41–42
Lo, B., 29, 65, 66, 69
Looman, C., 87, 88, 104, 148
Luce, J., 35, 36–37, 64
Lynn, J., 59, 70, 72, 73, 131, 142, 143

Maclean, H., 87, 88, 89, 148
Maddi, S., 57, 58
Maddox, P., 117, 128
Magno, J., 4, 129, 133
Malphurs, J., 91
Marcial, W., 20, 142
Marshall, P., 6
Marson, D., 48, 50
Martin, D., 16, 17, 154
Marwit, S., 152, 154
Matross, G., 34, 62
Mayo, D., 60, 63, 66

SUBJECT INDEX

195

Cost control
    hospice care and, 22–23
    vs. self-determination, 21–23
Criminal justice, 32
Criteria for competency, 41–45
Cruzan, Nancy Beth, 13, 33, 35, 58, 60,
    68–70, 77–78, 114
Cultural issues, 4, 6–7
    death with dignity in, 20–21
    youth oriented, death denying cultures
      and, 23

Danforth, John, 35
Death with dignity, 14, 17–21, 164, 167
    cultural issues in, 20–21
Death, perception of, 163–167
Decent minimum level of care, access to
    care and, 125
Decision making by patient, psychologist's
    role and, 153–154, 155
Deductive models of ethical decision mak-
    ing, 28–29
Defense-based denial, competency and, 44
Degenerative disease, 12, 14
Dehydration, terminal, 65–66
Dementia patients, 14, 50–51
Depression, 3, 85, 87, 150–151, 153
Descartes, Rene, 163
Developmentally disabled patients, compe-
    tency and, 52
Dignity conserving care, 19, 167
Dignity in dying (*See* death with dignity)
Distributive justice, 32
Do no harm principle vs. assisted suicide, 90
Do Not Intubate (DNI) orders, 57
Do Not Resuscitate (DNR) orders, 57, 67,
    72, 114, 136
Double effect principle, 62, 63–64
    ethical and legal issues in, 31, 37
Due care, voluntary euthanasia and, 104
Durable power of attorney for health care,
    69–70

Economic issues, 10
Effectiveness of advance directives, 70–73
Emancipated minors, competency and, 51
Embryonic stem cells, 12
End-of-life preparation at advanced stage of
    illness, system for, 143–146
Endostatin, 12

Epidemic diseases, 12
Ethical and legal issues, 27–53, 160
    advance directives and, 28
    assisted suicide and, 36–37, 89–90
    autonomy principle in, 29–30
    beneficence principle in, 30–31
    competency concept and, in informed
      consent, 38
    competency/incompetent patients
      and, informed consent, 39–52
    double effect principle in, 31, 37
    end of life decisions and, guiding prin-
      ciples of, 28–34
    Ethics Advisory Committee (EAC)
      in, 41
    informed consent and, 37–40
    insurance coverage and, 32–33
    justice principle in, 32–33
    legal bases for end of life decision in,
      34–40
    liberty interest concept in, 35
    living wills and, 35
    medical technology and, 27
    mercy principle in, 31
    models of ethical decision making,
      28–29
    natural death statutes in, 35
    nonmaleficence principle in, 31–32
    paternalism and, 30
    Patient Self-Determination Act
      (PSDA), 35–36
    process of ethical decision making in,
      33–34
    rationing of care and, 33
    refusal of life-sustaining treatment
      and, 34–36
    special patient populations and com-
      petency status in, 49–52
    voluntariness concept and, in
      informed consent, 38
Ethics Advisory Committee (EAC), 41, 78,
    148, 160–162
Eurotransplant Foundation, 119
Euthanasia, voluntary (*See also* assisted sui-
    cide), 101–106
    Initiative 119 (Washington) and, 101
    Netherlands and, 103–105
    Oregon Death with Dignity Act
      (ODDA), 101
    pro and con arguments for, 102–103
    Proposition 161 (California) and, 101
    refusal of treatment and, 61–62

MacArthur Treatment Competence Study, 48

Macroallocation of care, 117

Mature minor doctrine, competency and, 51

McGill Quality of Life Questionnaire (MQOL), 24–25, 26

Medicaid, 21, 123–126
    alternatives in care and, 139
    home care, 142

Medical progress/technology, 10–11, 23–24, 23
    ethical and legal issues in, 27
    prolonging life and, 110

Medicare, 17, 21, 123–126, 130
    alternatives in care and, 134, 139–141
    home care and, 142–143, 142

"Medicaring," 143

Mental status examination (MSE), 47

Mentally ill patients, competency and, 49–50

Mercy principle, in ethical and legal issues, 31

Microallocation of care, 117

Missoula-VITAS Quality of Life Index (MVQOLI), 25–26

Models of ethical decision making, 28–29

Mourning, stages of, 157–158

Natanson v. Kline, 37

National Hospice Study, 134, 135, 155

Natural death concept, 18–19

Natural death statutes, 35

Netherlands
    and assisted suicide, 97–99
    and voluntary euthanasia, 103–105

Nguyen, Ryan, 112–114

Nonmaleficence principle, in ethical and legal issues, 31–32

Nursing homes, 21, 138–140

NuTech movement, 92–94

Nutrition, withdrawal/withholding of, 57–58, 67

O'Connor, 64–65

Oregon and assisted suicide, 95–97

Oregon Basic Health Services Act, access to care and, 125

Oregon Death with Dignity Act (ODDA), 56, 95–97, 99–101, 132

Organ transplants, rationing of, 117–123

Organic-based test of competency, 44

Pain and Policy Studies Group, University of Wisconsin, 132

Pain control, 3, 19, 132–134, 151–152, 163–167
    and double effect principle in, 63–64

Pain: The Fifth Vital Sign, 133

Palliative care, 68, 85–86, 133–136
    assisted suicide and, 97
    psychologist's role and, 154–155, 156

Parkinson's disease, 14

Paternalism vs. autonomy principle, 30, 62

Patient Self-Determination Act (PSDA), 21–23, 35–36, 56, 69–70, 73, 77

Pearlman, Robert, 77

Perceptions of Disorder (POD), 48, 49

Physician-assisted suicide (*See* assisted suicide; euthanasia, voluntary)

Prescription drug laws, 131–132

President's Commission for the Study of Ethical Problems in Medicine, Biomedical, Behavioral Research, 160

Prior to progressive and life-threatening illness, 148–149

Process of ethical decision making, 33–34

Prolonged dying and quality of life, 13–14

Prolonging life, 10, 109–128
    AMA recommendations in, 113–114, 116
    Cruzan case in, 114
    defining "futile treatment" in, 112–114
    Do Not Resuscitate (DNR) orders and, 114
    futility debate and, 110–117
    Houston Bioethics Network and, 115
    medical technology and, 110
    organ transplants and, 117–123
    process for deciding "futile treatment", 114–117
    Quinlan case in, 114
    rationing of care and, 110, 117–123
    Veterans Health Administration (VHA) guidelines in, 116

Proposition 161 (California), voluntary euthanasia, 101

Psychologist's role, 147–162
    assisted suicide and, 154

ABOUT THE AUTHOR

Phillip M. Kleespies, PhD, was awarded his doctoral degree in clinical psychology from Clark University in 1971. He is the coordinator of emergency and urgent care services for psychology and has been appointed as director of a new behavioral health/crisis stabilization clinic that is being developed at the Boston campus of the VA Boston Healthcare System. Dr. Kleespies is a member of the Boston VA Ethics Advisory Committee and has written on issues related to ethics and the end-of-life choices available to patients who are terminally ill. He also has made numerous presentations and has written or edited publications on evaluating potential for suicidal and violent behavior and the impact of such patient behavioral emergencies on clinicians. He edited *Emergencies in Mental Health Practice: Evaluation and Management* (1998).

Dr. Kleespies is a diplomate in clinical psychology of the American Board of Professional Psychology and a fellow of the American Psychological Association (APA). He was the founding president of Section VII, Emergencies and Crises, of APA Division 12 (Society of Clinical Psychology) and is currently the treasurer of this section. He resides with his wife in Cambridge, Massachusetts.

So much
tissue form
w/o a real
integration of
psych & spiritual
issues!
The book shows
the emptiness
of a
scientific driven
psychology in
the context of the
liberal group
think.